The Undruggist: Book One

A Tale of Modern Apothecary and Wellness

Larry J. Frieders, RPh

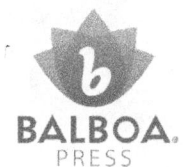

Copyright © 2010 by Larry J. Frieders, RPh

All rights reserved. No part of this book may be used or reproduced by any means, graphic, electronic, or mechanical, including photocopying, recording, taping or by any information storage retrieval system without the written permission of the publisher except in the case of brief quotations embodied in critical articles and reviews.

Balboa Press books may be ordered through booksellers or by contacting:

Balboa Press
A Division of Hay House
1663 Liberty Drive
Bloomington, IN 47403
www.balboapress.com
1-(877) 407-4847

Because of the dynamic nature of the Internet, any Web addresses or links contained in this book may have changed since publication and may no longer be valid. The views expressed in this work are solely those of the author and do not necessarily reflect the views of the publisher, and the publisher hereby disclaims any responsibility for them.

The author of this book does not dispense medical advice or prescribe the use of any technique as a form of treatment for physical, emotional, or medical problems without the advice of a physician, either directly or indirectly. The intent of the author is only to offer information of a general nature to help you in your quest for emotional and spiritual well-being. In the event you use any of the information in this book for yourself, which is your constitutional right, the author and the publisher assume no responsibility for your actions.

Any people depicted in stock imagery provided by Thinkstock are models, and such images are being used for illustrative purposes only.
Certain stock imagery © Thinkstock.

ISBN: 978-1-4525-0087-4 (sc)
ISBN: 978-1-4525-0089-8 (dj)
ISBN: 978-1-4525-0088-1 (e)

Library of Congress Control Number: 2010915328

Printed in the United States of America

Balboa Press rev. date: 11/17/2010

Contents

Foreword by Joel Frieders vii

Introduction – *Too Many People Take Too Many Drugs* ix
- How much is too much? xi
- Bad design or too much insult? xii
- Your medicine can harm ALL of us! xiii

Section One – Compounding; Art and Science 1
- A brief history of pharmacy 4
- One size does NOT fit all 5
- Wellness is more than "good enough" 6
- The Art and Science of Compounding is a Necessity 9

Section Two – Home Remedies and Common Sense 15

An Introduction to Home Remedies 17

Chapter One – Urinary Control 19
- The Urge to Urinate 19
- Four Simple Steps for Taking Urinary Control 21
- How to Kegel… 23
- What about women? 24

Chapter Two – Bad Breath 27
- Causes of most cases of bad breath… 28
- I'll wash your mouth out with soap! 29
- Rinse with water 30
- Bad breath from the belly… 31

Chapter Three – UTI's (Urinary Tract Infections) 33
- Warning: UTI's need to be treated 35
- Frequent UTI's 37

CHAPTER FOUR – SHAVING WITHOUT TEARS 39
- Shave with OIL. 40

CHAPTER FIVE – MY THROAT HURTS! 45
- Why does my throat hurt?. 45
- Get some relief… 47

CHAPTER SIX – WHAT?! THERE MUST BE SOMETHING WRONG WITH THE SCALE! 51
- Recommendations on weight loss… 52

SECTION THREE – HEALTHY CHOICES 59

INTRODUCTION – WELLNESS IS A CHOICE 61

CHAPTER ONE – WHAT "THEY" DON'T WANT YOU TO KNOW ABOUT VITAMINS. 63

CHAPTER TWO – SMOKING AND THE <u>REAL</u> "LITTLE BLUE PILL" . . .69

CHAPTER THREE – COUNTING TO TEN; THE "TEN DAY" RULE 75

CHAPTER FOUR – WATER, WATER EVERYWHERE…. 79

CONCLUSION 85

TESTIMONIAL. 93

Foreword by Joel Frieders

"Toss a man a fish and he'll eat for a few minutes, teach him how to use explosives and he'll be fishing in his own pond, eating fish off of diamond plates until he dies."

-Author Unknown

Growing up in a house with two pharmacist parents meant I didn't get away with a lot. I was only kept home from school when I was contagious or too ill to function normally. And while that didn't allow for a much desired mid-week sabbatical during high school, it did teach me an understanding of when my body was actually in need of healing or medical attention. Along with this understanding came a respect for time.

My dad would look at what hurt, make sure it wasn't broken, bleeding or inflamed and tell me to watch it for a few days.

Sure enough, a few days later I would either be on the road to recovery or have already forgotten about what had initially panicked me. I learned that my body was capable of healing itself in most situations, and by adding a medicine I didn't need or a doctor visit I could have avoided, I would usually make more of something than it deserved.

Larry J. Frieders, RPh

My father was notorious for saying "You're making a mountain out of a molehill!" whenever one of us made a dramatic production out of something that would be gone in a day or two.

It is this frame of mind that is missing from our society in 2010.

Every ailment has a medicine, every body part a specialist. Every problem has a reason, and those reasons are routinely treated with chemicals that create more problems than they solve. If we operated under a guise of personal restraint and held off on forcing our way into a doctor's office every time a red bump shows up on our child's forearm to demand an antibiotic, we might learn that our bodies are in fact the miraculous organisms of science fiction.

We've just been too busy whining to realize it.

Health is not a result of successful doctoring or prescribing, but a cumulative result of utilizing common sense, trusted experts and above all else, patience.

Our society needs this book now, more than ever.

JOEL FRIEDERS

Introduction –
Too Many People Take Too Many Drugs

Remember the '70's? All those psychedelic swirls? All that '60's hangover? The Beatles had broken up but continued to produce amazing music as individual artists. Even though The Eagles were "Takin' It Easy," as a nation we were still roiled by political and cultural debates. "Our Bodies, Ourselves" opened the eyes of many women – and more than a few men – to the truth about their own bodies.

Richard Nixon was President.

We all had more hair.

Remember?

I sure do. It was during the 70's that I became a health professional. At the time, those of us who cared about the well-being of our patients were alarmed by a phenomenon called "poly-pharmacy," which referred to the troubling situation in which an individual was taking multiple medications. As a pharmacist, I knew only too well that multiple medications exponentially increased the potential for adverse side effects.

Three medications at once seemed astonishingly – and almost always, unnecessarily – risky.

Pharmacists and health professionals were not alone in being troubled by the rise in medication overuse. My patients were concerned as well. People who had rarely taken anything stronger than the occasional aspirin tablet suddenly found multiple medicine bottles staring back at them when they opened their medicine cabinets.

I still remember the afternoon Mrs. Goldsmith came into my pharmacy, clutching a prescription she'd just received from her doctor. At the time, she was in her late seventies, self-sufficient, opinionated and no stranger to hardship.

"What's this, Mrs. Goldsmith?" I asked as she pushed the crumpled piece of paper across the counter to me.

Her lips tightened in an angry scowl. "Doctor says I have to take it," she spat out. She shook her head as I picked up the prescription and began to read it. "These darned pills. I can't hardly keep track of them all." She rolled her eyes and then furrowed her brow. "In the morning. In the evening. With food. On an empty stomach…it's ridiculous."

I had to agree with her. As her pharmacist, I knew she was already on a "water pill" for her high blood pressure and another for a thyroid condition. This additional prescription would make *three* medications she would have to take every day. "Let me give the doctor a call and see what I can find out," I told her.

"Would you?" she asked gratefully.

"Of course."

In another sign of how the times have changed, unlike today, her doctor got right on the phone when I called. After a few brief pleasantries, I voiced my concern about how these medications might interact. He listened considerately and acknowledged the concern but remained insistent that she take all three medications. In a small concession to the potential for danger, he altered the dosage of her blood pressure medication.

After our conversation, I hung up the phone and shook my head with the same kind of confusion I was sure Mrs. Goldsmith had felt. Three medications!

Looking back, my outrage seems almost quaint. If you would have told me when I first began my professional career that by the beginning of the 21st century that I would be hard-pressed to find someone *not* on at least three medications and that it would not be uncommon for someone to be taking as many as ten or even fifteen medications regularly I would have told you that you were out of your mind.

Heck, I'd have sworn to you that the Apocalypse would arrive first. Ten or fifteen medications? What could anyone possibly take so many medications *for*?

But that was before Big Pharma began developing medicines to solve every malady and complaint. Psychotropics. Statins. GERD medications. Creams for baldness. Arthritis medication. Pain medication. High Blood Pressure medication. Beta blockers. Calcium channel blockers. Allergy medications. Birth control pills. Erectile dysfunction medication. Hormone therapies. Ritalin. Antibiotics (too often for *viral* illnesses!) Daily baby aspirin. Diet pills. Over-the-counter cough medicine. St. John's Wort. On and on and on…

As we all know, a lot has changed in these past forty years. One thing that *hasn't* changed is our basic biology and physiology. Our bodies work pretty much the same as they did four thousand years ago, let alone forty.

- ### How Much Is Too Much?

Pharmacists and researchers have known for decades that three medications is the upper limit of what our bodies can tolerate with reasonable safety. Adding more than three medications to the mix increases the potential for serious adverse reactions. And yet, we have reached a point where the average person thinks nothing of taking multiple medications – both prescribed and over-the-counter. To them, powerful medications pose less risk than candy. In fact, they often think candy is *more* dangerous. Refined sugar and all…

People think of medication as benign. Even "harmless."

Those "fine print" inserts? Who can be bothered with all that technical stuff?

• BAD DESIGN OR TOO MUCH INSULT?

Something has gone very, very wrong in our "relationship" with the medications we take. Likewise, something has gone very wrong in our relationship with our own bodies. From where I stand, the need for so many medications to survive means one of two things – either we have been designed improperly, or our perfectly good bodies have been damaged. I reject out of hand that we have been improperly designed. Quite the contrary, I maintain that we are remarkable physical beings.

Our bodies are masterful examples of physiology and engineering. If they weren't, we would not have been able to survive – and thrive – in so many diverse and harsh environments for all these many thousands of years. Our bodies suffer insult and injury *and heal themselves.*

When given the chance, that is.

Our physiology has not changed in thousands upon thousands of years. What *has* changed is the pharmaceutical industry and our cultural (versus, biological) tolerance for medication. Now, I am not railing against the pharmaceutical industry *per se*. Medications are *important* and, when used appropriately, save lives and improve well-being. Many, many people benefit from the kinds of medications that are being created and produced every day.

"Big Pharma" is *a* problem but it is not *the* problem. The truth is, *we* are all the problem. We have lost our perspective about what medications can and cannot do; what they *should* and should not do.

Our bodies have not changed, not in a very long time. Yet we desperately *believe* we need these many medications to survive. Well, if our bodies are as well-designed as I insist then the obvious implication is that we have damaged our perfectly well-designed bodies so that we need these medications. I think this is both true and untrue. In some ways, we have created a world that hurls insults at our bodies unlike any we have ever known. But the sad irony is that *over*-medicating ourselves actually results in *more* damage to our bodies, not more healing. The potential harm that all these medications represent is significant — to individuals and to communities.

- ### YOUR MEDICINE CAN HARM *ALL* OF US!

The immediate potential for danger is to the individual taking all those ten or fifteen medications. But just as alarming is the fact that the medication YOU take can harm ME!

No medication is absorbed completely — not in the process of producing it and not in your use of it. A percentage of the medication you take is excreted from your body. That finds its way into our community waste system and, eventually, into our water supply. So, as a result of all this medication, our communal water supply has been polluted by medications and metabolites. We drink that water and unwittingly — and without choice — we ingest those medications.

We are not the only ones. Every living creature depends on water to survive. Other creatures drink that water too, creatures that very often end up in our food supply, adding to our ingesting of these medicines.

As a result, whether by choice or not, we are taking *even more* pharmaceuticals than we intend. Pregnant women are ingesting medicines not designed for them, many of which are able to penetrate the protective barrier of the placenta and affect their unborn children. Toddlers, whose bodies are in their earliest stages of development are introduced to the same medicines that eighty year olds are taking.

I am a licensed pharmacist. I value the potential benefit that medication holds for good health. I also know the potential danger these same medications present. As a result, for many years I have considered myself to be in "recovery" as a pharmacist.

No, I have never had a problem with abuse. I am recovering pharmacist in the sense that I am recovering from the mindset that proclaims that "if a little medicine is good for you, a lot must be better." I'm a recovering pharmacist because I have long become alarmed by the potential risks posed by the very medications supposedly designed to heal us. I am a recovering pharmacist because I think we can do a better job of taking care of ourselves.

Once I became convinced that the risk was real, I could not in good conscience continue business as usual, to work in a "common" pharmacy – which is, in truth, nothing more than an outlet in the chain of pharmaceutical dispensing. I have maintained my pharmacy license but I cannot participate in a process that I know in my heart to be excessive, wrong-headed and dangerous.

We – physicians, pharmacists, pharmaceutical companies, patients – have lost our way. We have focused on the medicine rather than the patient. Our focus is medicine-centered rather than patient/healing-centered. It is past time to shift that focus from medicine and marketing back to the patient and healing.

Health care is a science and an art. One can disagree and engage in the important discussion about the balance between the two but we should all be able to agree on one thing – when medicine and the delivery of pharmaceuticals becomes primarily a business, patients and healing suffer. I object to the modern system of excess drug use, the one where pharmacists can make a living only by selling more drugs.

When I started in this business, the most common title for us was "Druggist", the professional outside the doctor's office who helped his customers achieve the health they wanted, and did so in a gentle, natural manner that supported and respected the true art of medicine. The doctor and the druggist were a team. Most of that has been abandoned in favor of a quick diagnosis and an even quicker prescription for the latest drug. The old title symbolized something special. Let's make the effort to rekindle trust in the true benefits of medicines. Until that time, I remain Larry Frieders, The Un-Druggist.

It's time to get back to the art of relieving suffering.

It's time to get back to the science of healing.

Section One – Compounding; Art and Science

An elderly man leads a young boy by the hand through the dusty, crooked streets of an old village. The boy constantly lags behind.

"Come," the elderly man urges the boy. His voice is gentle but his tone suggests urgency. He tugs on the boy's hand.

The boy plods along but it is not easy. He has not been well. A fever raged in him for several days. After the fever broke, he was unable to hold any food down. Now, he is weak and unable to help with his chores.

"I can't," the boy complains in a soft voice.

The elderly man stops and considers the boy. His eyes are compassionate. He doesn't know what best to do. He is old. Finally, despite his age, he lifts the boy and places him on his shoulders, carrying him the last few blocks to the shop he is looking for.

Inside, the air is cool and still. A man looks up with a questioning gaze.

"The boy is sick," the elderly man says as he sets him down.

The man comes over and places his palm against the boy's forehead. He speaks to the boy and the old man. Then he gathers some leaves and powders from behind a counter and mashes them together with a stone pestle. He then combines the powder into some warm water and gives it to the boy to drink.

"Take him home," he says to the old man. "He will be better tomorrow..."

Larry J. Frieders, RPh

In our collective imagination, we hold dear the image of the healer, someone who is capable of assessing a person's malady and then, by intuition and knowledge, bring together the various herbs and medicines – in the exact amounts – that will bring about relief and healing. This shared image is not the result of some Hollywood fantasy but the reality of how the healing arts have existed for thousands of years.

- *A BRIEF HISTORY OF PHARMACY...*

There are 3rd or 4th century AD Indian Ayurvedic texts that refer to compilation of medical substances. Reaching even further back into the shadows of our shared pre-history, these texts themselves refer to Sushruta, considered to be a medical sage from the 6th century BC. Eight thousand years ago, the art of making medicine was recognized and documented.

The Sumerians (remember those clay tablets with the earliest forms of writing that we all learned about in school?) recorded medicine prescriptions in cuneiform. The Egyptians maintained their knowledge of medicines on papyruses. The ancient Chinese had the "Recipes for 52 Ailments," a text of specific remedies that was first discovered in a tomb that had been sealed in 168 BC.

Pedanius Dioscorides, a Greek physician, wrote a five-volume encyclopedia about "medical substances" which formed the foundation upon which the great scholars of Islam built their scientific understanding during the Golden Age of Islam.

An ancient pharmacy in Turkey was designated by a stone sign showing a tripod, a mortar, and a pestle.

Islam saw incredible growth in knowledge and understanding during the 9th and 10th centuries AD. Studies of botany and chemistry led to the development of modern pharmacology. Processes of sublimation and distillation were pioneered. Al-Biruni wrote, *Kitab al-Saydalah*

(The Book of Drugs,) in which he delineated the properties of drugs and outlined the role of pharmacy and the functions and duties of the pharmacist – over a thousand years ago!

By the 12th century, shops devoted to pharmacy began to appear in Europe. And a handful of pharmacies from those early years are still open today. Healing *was* pharmacology. The apothecary was the healer in most cultures, giving medical advice and care that are now performed by specialists. He was the person who formulated and dispensed medical material to physicians, surgeons or directly to patients. (Wikipedia, *History of Pharmacy*)

Japan, Baghdad, Africa, South America – it is no wonder that, with this long history of healing that found realization in every corner of the world, our collective image of the "healer" is someone who has been called apothecary, chemist, pharmacist or compounder.

- ### ONE SIZE DOES *NOT* FIT ALL

Throughout history, pharmacy compounding has been the link between patient and healing. Sadly, what we actually see in our modern world often bears little resemblance to that ancient, wise image. In our modern world, medicines are pre-packaged, one-size fits all. The determination about that "one-size" has a much, or more, to do with marketing than it does to healing. Regardless, when it comes to health, one size does *not* fit all. And, most importantly, when it comes to your health, there is only one size that matters – yours.

Complicating the "one-size fits all" mindset is a mentality that seems to suggest that each and every health issue is nothing more than a "problem" to be "solved" and that every problem, malady or discomfort can be solved readily by simply taking a pill.

Heart not functioning efficiently? Take a pill.

Feeling down? Take a pill.

Runny nose from seasonal allergies? Take a pill.

Having trouble concentrating on your studies? Take a pill.

Need to lose a couple of pounds? Well, you get the idea.

The mentality that all that ails us can be quickly and easily addressed by taking a pill subverts the basic truth that if we're taking medicines it is because we have done harm to our body (rather than there being a flaw in the design). Taking a pill to "solve" the harm fails to address the underlying harm. Therefore, real healing cannot fully take place.

Make no mistake; there are some maladies for which medication *is* the answer. But often, healing involves *all* the various ways that we can to allow our bodies to self-correct the underlying harm. Medication simply provides the temporary support to help this process occur.

- ## Wellness is more than "good enough"

A couple of weeks ago, a middle-aged man came into The Compounder Pharmacy. He was the epitome of the phrase, "sick as a dog." He was pale. His skin was moist. He walked gingerly, as if walking hurt. He was coughing. He was a mess.

"What do you have for a cold?" he asked me.

"Hot tea and a couple of days in bed," I said.

He shook his head. "No. I have to go to work. Got a presentation." He began to cough violently. "I feel terrible…"

I felt bad for the guy. He sounded even worse than he looked.

"I just need something so I'm good enough to go to work…," he said.

Although I sympathized with his desire to meet his obligations and responsibilities, I also knew that he epitomized the "quick fix" view of medicine and pharmaceuticals. "Just make me better." Or, more correctly, "Make *it* better." As if whatever ails us is separate from us.

Until we understand, accept and embrace that we are not simply the sum of all our parts, that there is a wholeness that *is* us, then we will continue to objectify our ailments and maladies, turning them into a "problem" that must be "solved," preferably by a pill or something equally tolerable.

We need to *allow ourselves* to get better (versus, *make ourselves* better.) In the process, we should avoid exposing others to our illnesses.

The truth is our bodies successfully overcome the vast majority of our ailments. Medicines can help but we still need to support our bodies in doing what they were designed to do. If we are sick, we still need to rest. We still need to drink plenty of hot fluids.

Medicines can have an important role to play in healing. But that role should not be independent of the body self-healing. Rather, it should be in concert with it. Pre-dosed, pre-packaged medicines are almost always overkill because they are not tailored to an individual's needs.

Traditional pharmacy has always been clear about the need to tailor medicine to the needs of specific ailments and individuals. This is why traditional pharmacies compounded medicines, rather than simply dispense bottles of pre-filled and pre-dosed medicine product. In the past, compounding *was* pharmacy. Throughout history, pharmacists compounded drugs for patients as they were prescribed by physicians.

A brief timeline of the history of pharmacy in the United States traces this history and where it shifted:

- In 1820, the U.S. Pharmacopeia established monographs for pharmacy compounding in the United States;

- In 1906, the U.S. Pure Food and Drug Act established the *U.S. Pharmacopoeia* and *National Formulary* as two of the official compendia of standards for pharmaceuticals in the United States;

- In the early 1900s, however, the pharmaceutical industry began manufacturing most drugs and dosage forms for patients;

- The U.S. Food and Drug Administration (FDA) was established with the passage of the Federal Food, Drug and Cosmetic Act of 1938 to develop and enforce standards for manufactured drugs;

- During the mid-1900s with the large effort by the pharmaceutical industry in providing numerous strengths and dosage forms for drugs, the need for compounding diminished;

- Since the late 1900s, however, a lot has changed and the pharmaceutical industry no longer supplies all the medications needed by patients. As a result, pharmacy compounding has experienced tremendous growth.

Although the history and need for compounding should be self-evident, there have been detractors who have demanded that the FDA exert even greater control over compounding. However, the FDA has been reluctant to do this, recognizing the importance of, and need for, pharmacy compounding. The same respect has been extended by the Supreme Court and the U.S. Congress; each has recognized the contribution of pharmacy compounding to modern health care today.

Oversight and enforcement of compounding exist at the state level. State Boards of Pharmacy have been established to enforce the components of these acts as they relate to pharmacy. This balance is as it should be. The FDA was created to enforce requirements on the pharmaceutical industry, not the practice of pharmacy.

Unfortunately, the FDA has expanded its "reach" in recent years and has begun to overstep its original enforcement mandate. Complicating the situation, some pharmacists have blurred the line by practicing in a "gray area" between compounding and manufacturing. Going forward, it is important that this gray area get clarified by the State Boards of Pharmacy.

That said, the need for compounding not only remains strong but it is growing stronger.

When the pharmaceutical industry began manufacturing a myriad of drugs and dosages on a large scale in the early 1900s, the need for compounding seemed to diminish. For a good part of the past century, the pharmaceutical industry addressed the needs of most patients fairly adequately. However, during the last part of the century, a great deal began to change and the pharmaceutical industry no longer met the needs of a great many patients.

- ## THE ART AND SCIENCE OF COMPOUNDING IS A NECESSITY

Compounding has become vital again for some of the following reasons:

1. Limited Dosage Strengths. The pharmaceutical industry maximizes profits by limiting the variation of the medicines it manufactures. This means that it produces only limited strengths of drugs. As I have noted before, one size does *not* fit all. It is often *necessary* to change the strength of a drug for individual patients. The only way to do that is by compounding.

2. Limited Dosage Forms. The pharmaceutical industry supplies only limited dosage forms; generally an oral solid (tablet or capsule) and/or injection. These forms are adequate for most adults – and again, to maximize profits – but they fail to address the needs of children, premature infants, the elderly, and special needs patients. In fact, Congress has made it possible for the industry to obtain additional patent protection if they manufacture a pediatric (children's) form of the drug, but most companies still do not do this

because it is not economically feasible for them; therefore, compounding is necessary.

3. Home Health Care. As we baby boomers age, we want to stay in our homes even as our health begins to fail us. That means home health care. However, home healthcare often requires compounded medications. For example, patients who have had colon surgery require total parenteral nutrition (intravenous fats, sugars, and amino acids) post-operatively. These patients cannot be satisfactorily medicated or sustain a nutritional status needed for healing with manufactured dosage forms.

4. Hospice and Palliative Care Patients. End-of-life therapy involves the compounding of many, many different and unique dosage forms to allow patients to live out their lives free of pain and discomfort. Many people in hospice care are unable to swallow medications or do not have the muscle mass required to receive multiple injections each day. For these patients, compounded medications for oral inhalation, nasal administration, topical/transdermal, and rectal use are necessary.

5. Discontinued Drugs. Motivated by profit, the pharmaceutical industry has discontinued thousands of drug products over the past 25 years. Despite not being profitable for the pharmaceutical industry, these products were often very effective. The only way they can now be made available to patients is through pharmacy compounding.

6. Drug Shortages. Drug manufacturing relies on bulk drug chemicals, which are often imported for the U.S. pharmaceutical industry and for compounding. Like any commodity, these chemicals are sometimes subject to shortages and unavailability for any number of reasons. When commercially manufactured drugs become unavailable, in many cases they can be compounded to help "bridge the gap" until the commercial product returns to the market.

7. Intravenous Admixtures in Hospitals. Many, if not most, of the lifesaving intravenous drugs given in hospitals and clinics are compounded. This saves the hospital personnel time and the patient multiple injections or administrations. It is hard to imagine being in the hospital without intravenous admixtures being available.

8. Orphan Drugs. When physicians prescribe drugs that are not on the market, they may be available as orphan drugs, either commercially or compounded.

9. Special Patient Populations. Included here would be *pain management* patients, *bioidentical hormone replacement therapy (BHRT)* patients, *sports injury* patients (professional, collegiate, Olympic and other amateur athletes), *dental* patients, *dermatological* patients, *environmentally and cosmetic sensitive* patients, as well as other patients who are being treated successfully with compounded medications prescribed by physicians. Specialty compounded drugs for eye surgery, bone surgery, etc. would not be available. *Cancer treatment* almost always involves compounded "cocktails", or mixtures of cancer drugs that would be unavailable if they could not be compounded.

10. New Therapeutic Approaches. If a physician desires to use a medication that is successfully used in other countries but is not commercially available here, that physician can prescribe a compounded formulation of the medication for patients. An FDA-approved oral therapy prescribed as a topical gel for arthritis treatment to avoid gastric bleeding could reduce the overall cost of healthcare by avoiding hospitalization from a gastric bleed.

11. Clinical Studies. Pharmacists compound drugs that are not commercially available that are used in various clinical studies.

12. Nuclear Compounding. A radioactive source is "tagged" to a compound that circulates throughout the body and

eventually concentrates in the organ under exploration. With over 100 different types of nuclear procedures performed every day, the most commonly performed procedure is organ imaging; to determine blood flow and function of the heart, blockage of the gallbladder, measure lungs for respiratory and blood-flow problems, bones for fracture, infection, arthritis or tumor, bleeding of the bowel, locate the presence of infection, measure thyroid function, and to determine the presence or spread of cancer.

13. Veterinary Compounding. Animals can be grouped into various categories, including small, large, herd, exotic, and companion groups. There are actually relatively few medications available for animals, and those medications that are available are for specific species and diseases. In most cases, for an animal to be satisfactorily treated, a compounded medication may be necessary.

Pharmacy compounding is necessary for many patient populations. Without pharmacy compounding, children would not be able to receive necessary medications in many of the forms they need - syrups, elixirs, suspensions, and emulsions. Parents who have had to fight losing battles with children to take their medication know that medicine in gummy bears, and popsicles make taking medications palatable for children. Compounding makes these forms possible. Elderly patients would not have access to new dosage forms to make it easier to take their medications. Hospitalized patients, without compounding, would have multiple drugs administered one at a time rather than in a single intravenous delivery.

Many patients have adverse reactions to medications *not* because they are allergic to the medication itself but because they are allergic to a preservative, dye, flavor, or other ingredient in a commercial product. Without compounding, these patients would not have access to beneficial medications.

It seems clear that pharmacy compounding is a vital part of making sure that the right medicine, in the right dose and the right form gets to the right patient.

Pharmacy compounding and common sense could go a long way toward healing and wellness.

Section Two – Home Remedies and Common Sense

An Introduction to Home Remedies

What was it that Dorothy said at the end of "The Wizard of Oz"? Something about, if she ever wanted to look for something ever again she knew she didn't have to look any further than her own backyard? I think the world is a wonderful place and a good deal larger than one's backyard. But there was real wisdom in Dorothy's realization. How often do we assume that the "answer" to our questions can only be found by searching far from home? Or, when it comes to addressing our various ailments, how often do we assume that relief can only be found in a pill or manufactured medication?

One of the great lessons I've learned as a "recovering pharmacist" is that our bodies' natural state is wellness. When we are unwell, our bodies *naturally* try to rectify the situation. That is, our bodies try to heal themselves.

If wellness is our goal, then the task is to support our bodies' natural inclination to heal. In which case, often, the best advice a pharmacist can give is to *not* take a formulated medication but rather, to find the solution a bit closer to home.

Chapter One – Urinary Control

- ### The Urge to Urinate

Not long ago, I went to a college football game with my friend Bob. He and I went to high school together. Even though we only see each other every couple of years, I consider him one of my best friends. We were both excited about this particular game because his son was playing, finishing up his senior year as a starter.

There was a lot riding on this particular game. It was Homecoming. Rival teams were playing. A league championship and bragging rights were involved. As befitted a game with so much on the line, it was a well-played contest from start to finish.

Several times during the game, Bob got up and asked me if I wanted anything – a beer, a hot dog, peanuts. I'd never known him to be so focused on snacks and goodies, but it was nice to have constant flow of food to accompany the great game.

"I'll get it," I told Bob, one time when he started to get up.

"No, no," he insisted. "I've got it."

He was getting up and down through the game, even into the fourth quarter. I was shocked when he got up with less than a minute to play and ambled up the stadium steps. But then the crowd cheered and my attention was turned back to the field where a tremendous running play put the team in the position to kick a last-second – and potential game-winning – field goal.

Bob returned just after the field goal went through the uprights.

"Did I miss anything?" he asked.

I looked at him, surprised. "Did you miss anything? That was an amazing finish. Are you all right?"

He shrugged. Then he smiled sheepishly. "You know what that commercial says, 'Always find yourself going…'" he said.

I knew only too well what the commercial said. As much as anything else, it had created a demand for its drug to treat benign prostatic hypertrophy (BPH) – the enlargement of the prostate, which often results in various urinary symptoms including the urge to constantly urinate.

"Hey, it happens to all of us, right?" he said, turning the question into a statement.

While it was true that most men experience prostate growth as they age, urinary symptoms are *not* necessarily the fate of most men. As we were leaving the stadium, I suggested that he see his doctor to rule out any serious condition that could cause his symptoms and then, assuming there was no serious underlying condition, to see me.

The answer to the "urge" to urinate is not necessarily a prescription but rather four simple steps that will return control to you. The fact is most men do *not have to experience* urinary symptoms. Of course, you'd never know that from the radio and television advertising for manufactured medication.

On the drive home from the football game, a radio ad proclaimed that "one out of every two men will have urinary problems after they're forty years old".

I rolled my eyes. "That's ridiculous," I said.

The announcer clearly didn't think so. He went on to point out ominously that, "symptoms never go away on their own…"

Bunk.

These scare tactics only confuse and complicate wellness. The truth is, except in extremely rare situations, any man can do these four, simple things to regain control. Four, simple things. Which is a lot better than taking medications or, worse, allowing uncomfortable symptoms to dictate how you will live your life.

- *Four Simple Steps for Taking Urinary Control*

The first step is counterintuitive – **Drink more water**.

When I suggested that to Bob he looked at me like I was out of my mind. "Hey, I'm going *too much* and you want me to drink *more*?"

Although it may seem counterproductive to drink more water when you are making multiple trips to the bathroom, it actually makes perfect sense once you understand how your body "knows" it's time to urinate. Nerves in the bladder and sphincter initiate the urge when the bladder is filled and when the urine is too concentrated. When you don't hydrate enough, your body thinks it needs to urinate when it doesn't!

How much fluid is enough? A good rule of thumb is one ounce of liquid (preferably, water!) for every two pounds of body weight. So a 200 pound man should drink about 100 ounces of fluid each day – a little over 3 quarts.

The second step is to **use a quality brand of saw palmetto and/or pygeum daily**, as directed on the bottle. Supplements are very useful because they do what their name implies – they "supplement" your body as it seeks its natural state of wellness. You should keep in mind that with supplements, quality is often directly associated with cost. You probably don't need to purchase the most expensive, but avoid the lowest priced ones.

BPH – benign, troubling <u>and</u> treatable!

In addition to these two methods, the third step you should consider is **the application of a small amount of progesterone cream 6 days a week** – most do best when they take a little time off every so often, once a week works best for me. You might associate progesterone with women but men have it as well – although in smaller amounts. BPH is associated with testicular function. Progesterone seems to have obvious benefit in relieving symptoms of BPH then. A dose of about 10mg applied to thin skin areas, such as the scrotum or inner arms, Monday through Saturday should do the trick.

Go to our website, www.thecompounder.com for more specific product information.

Finally, the fourth step is one that might make the *most* sense to you. **Exercise.**

Kegel – a noun and a verb!

After all, the bladder is a muscular organ. It makes sense that strengthening the muscles associated with the bladder will give you more control. Kegel exercises are most beneficial to bladder control focuses on a particular muscle group, the pubococcygeus muscle, or PC muscle. The PC muscle is a hammock-like muscle, found in both sexes, that stretches from the pubic bone to the coccyx (tail bone) forming the floor of the pelvic cavity and supporting the pelvic organs. It controls urine flow and contracts during orgasm. (Wikipedia)

Like any other muscle, the PC muscles can lose tone and get flabby. A flabby PC is NOT a terminal situation. As long as you are breathing and peeing, you can strengthen your PC muscles. The sooner you start doing Kegels... the quicker you'll see results. It may take a week. It may take a month. But the benefits of strengthening your PC muscles are tremendous. Personally, I cannot imagine why anyone *wouldn't* exercise his PC muscles – everyday.

In addition to controlling urine, your PC muscles control the flow of semen, the firmness of your erection and the shooting power of your ejaculation. (Did I mention I can't imagine why anyone wouldn't exercise these muscles?)

Exercising the PC muscles is simple and easy. It's safe. Discreet. You can exercise your PC muscles while sitting at your desk – at work!

- ## How to Kegel...

First, you need to locate your PC muscles. The easiest way to find them is to stop your flow of urine mid-flow next time you go to the bathroom. The muscles you use to stop the flow... those are your PC muscles. Once you've isolated them, practice flexing them and feeling exactly where they are located – it is easy to overcompensate for weak muscles by using the abdominals, buttocks or thighs. These must all stay relaxed when doing Kegel exercises.

Don't overdo it. I know it is tempting to throw yourself into something head on, especially when it could result in better sex. However, like any other muscle you exercise when you're working out, you need to give it some time to heal between sessions. This means regular rests and not overdoing it. If you follow the exercise schedule as you see fit, you should soon be great. Just listen to your body. It knows what it's talking about!

- ## WHAT ABOUT WOMEN?

That's a fine list of suggestions for men who "go" too much, but what about women with the same kind of symptoms? They don't have issues with a prostate that swells and pinches off the urine flow. Women are clearly different, but the problems are often the result of similar things. Women need to look at three specific areas to address urinary control.

The first is **proper hydration**.

The water issue is important, regardless of your gender. Many of us don't drink enough to keep ourselves properly hydrated. Water is available through a number of sources and they all contribute to our overall hydration. Be careful, though, about your sources. Caffeine is a diuretic. It stimulates urine flow. Alcohol can also be a diuretic. While you might be taking in sufficient liquids, your own body might be eliminating much of the total water that it needs for optimal function. I'm not suggesting anyone totally eliminate coffee, tea, or "adult beverages", but be mindful that they don't fulfill the body's need for water and hydration.

Secondly, **hormone balance** is vital to both genders.

The condition of our environment places practically everyone into a state of estrogen dominance – a situation in which we exhibit symptoms associated with excess estrogen while our estrogen levels fall below the normal ranges. The reason for this apparent conflict is that we are exposed to many substances in the environment that act like estrogens in our bodies, yet don't show up in standard hormone tests. Substances like pesticides and plasticizers can often trick the body into operating as if it has excess estrogen.

Progesterone to the rescue! Most women do well by applying small amounts of progesterone topical cream. They apply the dose once or twice daily – and are careful to skip a few days each month – an effort to somewhat mimic the natural rise and fall of progesterone during the menstrual cycle. Have questions about the use of Progesterone Cream? Visit my website and I can provide you with answers to all of your questions. Remember, visit www.thecompounder.com and search 'progesterone cream'.

Now, here's another apparent conflict.

Women who have urinary problems – leaking when coughing or laughing – might benefit from very small amounts of an estrogen cream. Many of our customers have benefitted by applying 0.1ml of a weak estrogen cream to their vaginal area one to three times a week. A doctor needs to write a prescription – estriol 0.05% is a good one. A compounder can make this into a gentle cream and dispense it in a device that makes dosing easy and accurate. It seems that vaginally applied estriol or estradiol works locally to strengthen and tone the muscles that control urine flow.

The key is in using small amounts. More is not better.

Finally, **exercise** needs to be a priority. The Kegel exercises are important for women – just as for men. If you're applying an estrogen cream to help tone muscles, it is a good plan to exercise those muscles. The exercise is the same for women as for men. Just SQUEEZE – HOLD – RELEASE – REPEAT.

Chapter Two – Bad Breath

There is a multi-million dollar industry dedicated to one thing and one thing alone – to convincing you that, 1) you have bad breath and, 2) their product is the very thing you need to do something about it.

How many first kisses have been ruined by the fear of bad breath?

How many relationships grounded before they ever developed because of this fear?

The reality is, people *do* have bad breath. But it is not a terrible thing and it is fairly easy to address – without going to great lengths or expense, or ruining your teeth by constantly chewing gum!

Bad Breath is also known as "halitosis." Most cases of bad breath begin in the mouth itself. Sometimes, bad breath is caused by a sulfur compound produced by bacteria. Dead and dying bacterial cells release this smelly sulfur compound. Sulfur products can bond – or stick – to the tissues lining the mouth. This creates an unpleasant odor that is also difficult to remove. People who suffer from gum disease (periodontitis) often have bad breath because bacteria (there's that bacteria again!) accumulates in areas that are not cleaned easily, such as deep pockets around teeth.

- **CAUSES OF MOST CASES OF BAD BREATH...**

While most cases of bad breath begin in the mouth, there are other causes that should be considered (and which need to be addressed by a doctor.)

- infections
- diabetes mellitus (sweet/alcohol)
- kidney failure (can produce a fishy odor)
- malfunction of the liver
- disorders of metabolism, and even fasting.

If you have treated the potential source of bad breath in the mouth and it still continues… it's time to speak with your doctor to rule out some other, more serious causes.

However, if your bad breath, like the vast majority of people with bad breath, originates in your mouth, there are some very simple natural remedies that should correct the situation.

Begin with good oral hygiene. Brush your teeth at least twice daily – and be sure to brush your teeth, your gums and your tongue. Use a soft brush and don't press too hard. Be gentle. You can damage the tissue of your teeth and gums, scrape cells off and cause small amounts of bleeding. Irritating the teeth and gums can cause swelling and separation of the gums from the tooth. That's where bacteria can hide – and create bad breath!

Choose your toothpaste carefully. Most commercial toothpastes contain harsh substances, such as silica (like fine sand), chemical sweeteners, sodium laurel sulfate, and preservatives. These can irritate sensitive tissue – and cause the same damage as brushing too hard.

Another common ingredient in most toothpaste is fluoride. It is a very toxic substance and it is irritating to the oral area. It is very good at preventing tooth decay but it can also do harm. Fluorine is a member of the same chemical family as chlorine (the chemical that's added to water to disinfect it); but is even more toxic. Exposing sensitive oral tissue to toxic substances irritates them, causing swelling. Just as with hard brushing, this creates pockets between the gums and teeth where bacteria can grow.

So, in addition to a soft bristle toothbrush, you should consider a gentler cleaner. Rather than a commercial toothpaste, you might consider regular baking soda. Simply, dampen your soft bristle toothbrush and sprinkle on some baking soda. Brush as usual. (Just don't stick your damp toothbrush into the box of soda. That's messy and unsanitary.)

- *I'LL WASH YOUR MOUTH OUT WITH SOAP!*

Who did not hear this threat when they were growing up, "If you use that language I'll wash your mouth out with soap!"?

Could there be a more humiliating punishment than that? And if you ever actually suffered the indignity of the punishment, you probably still remember how awful the soap tasted... so, you'll probably think I'm crazy to suggest to you that you wash your mouth out with soap. But that's exactly what I'm suggesting. And don't worry about the taste. It's only the back part of your tongue that's sensitive to the bitterness of the soap. Up front, and around all your teeth, you'll hardly notice the taste at all.

As it turns out, regular bar soap is a *great* tooth cleaner. Wet your toothbrush and apply the soap. But don't rub your toothbrush across the bar of soap itself. That's messy and unsanitary. You can "suds up" and apply the suds to your toothbrush or, even better, use a new product made especially for brushing – tooth soap. Place a couple of pieces of shredded soap on the damp brush and start brushing. Be gentle and clean all surfaces, for a full two minutes. Rinse the suds with water.

You should always rinse your mouth well after brushing, two to three times. Anything left behind in the oral cavity can be a source of odor.

So,

- Brush well.
- Brush often.
- And rinse, rinse, rinse.

Remember, don't be too rough. You don't want to damage the tissue in your mouth or cause bleeding. If you find that your gums bleed when you brush, you either need to see a dentist, or you need to be much more gentle on your gums.

The Compounder Pharmacy carries a number of tooth soaps. A visit to the website will tell you all you need to know about them.

- *RINSE WITH WATER*

When you rinse, rinse with plain water, not a flavored, sweetened mouthwash. Anything other than water just puts things back into the mouth you've just cleaned away. If you feel you must use a mouthwash after brushing, be sure to rinse well with water afterwards.

A clean oral cavity is an odor free oral cavity.

If "clean" isn't the freshness you're looking for and you'd like to add just a hint of mint, use drops or sprays that don't contain sugar. Try a breath freshener that contains pure essential oils, stevia and filtered water, something with no preservatives, glycerin or contaminating substances.

- ## BAD BREATH FROM THE BELLY...

Sometimes, bad breath is the result of what's in our stomachs rather than what's in our mouths. The question is, Is there a natural bad breath remedy for the times when we eat? This depends on how our food is handled once it gets to our stomach. There are bacteria in the digestive tract that help prepare food for absorption. Some of it is good for us and some isn't. Most of the time the good and harmful bacteria are in balance and everything works smoothly. However, it is very common for slight imbalance to occur, and the amount of good bacteria can fall.

Without an adequate supply of the good bacteria, some foods are converted to chemicals that contribute to bad breath. Restoring bacterial balance to your stomach is quite easy. A source of good bacteria is available, called probiotics: lactobacillus, bifidus, or acidophilus.

A daily dose of probiotics does wonders for keeping mouth odor under control. The good bacteria in the probiotics helps you fully digest food so that they do not retain their odors. Using probiotics can even reduce the sulfur odors that follow eating spices and strong foods like onions, shallots and garlic.

The bacteria in probiotics are natural, so using them as a natural bad breath remedy is a healthy idea.

There are many brands of probiotics, some better than others. Look for one that provides around 10 billion colony forming units of good bacteria in each dose. You'll want fresh probiotics and the freshest are kept in the refrigerator section of the store. We use Florajen 3. Look for it on our website, www.thecompounder.com.

Chapter Three –
UTI's (Urinary Tract Infections)

No, UTI's are *not* related to UFO's. And, to the people who suffer from them – primarily women – they are no laughing matter. UTI's are *Urinary Tract Infections* or, Bladder Infections. They tend to affect women more than men because of the relative shortness of a female's urethra – the tube that carries urine from the bladder. And they can come on quite suddenly.

Not terribly long ago, we took a weekend "road trip" with another couple when Ellen felt an urgent need to use the restroom.

"Just another few miles to the next rest area," I said, glancing at her in the rear view mirror. Seeing the distress on her face, I asked if she was feeling okay.

She grimaced. "I'll be all right," she said.

"How far is it?" she asked, a couple of minutes later.

"I don't think very far," I said. "Are you all right? Do you want me to pull over?"

She didn't answer. Howard, her husband, seemed to understand that something was more of a problem than a simple "bathroom stop." "What's the matter?" he asked, leaning closer to her.

Rather than answer, she leaned a bit forward. "Maybe you should pull over at the first chance," she said. "Preferably someplace with a bit of privacy."

Fortunately, there was a turn-off less than a mile later. Ellen rushed out of the car and ran toward a small outcropping of trees and brush. Howard sat awkwardly and shrugged, not knowing what to think. Patricia went walking in Ellen's direction.

We sat in an awkward silence for a moment or two.

"Everything was fine this morning?"

"Yes. We'd been looking forward to spending time with you guys for a while."

A few moments later, Ellen and Patricia were walking back toward the car. Ellen was mortified that she had needed to have me pull over so she could urinate 'on the side of the road,' she noted, her cheeks reddening.

Patricia laughed, immediately putting Ellen at ease. "If I count the number of times we've had to pull over…" Then her voice grew more comforting. "Bladder infections can sneak up on you."

Ellen nodded. "I should have known when I felt some burning this morning," she said, sounding angry with herself.

After a certain age, there are few women who have not suffered from at least one bout of UTI in their lives and are familiar with the burning sensation and powerful and frequent urge to urinate. Often, there is a bit of blood in the urine along with a strong smell.

Ellen remained quiet when we got back in the car. Even though the rest area was only another three miles up the road, we stopped in.

"Maybe I should just give my doctor a call," she said apologetically. "He might be able to call a prescription in to a local pharmacy."

Although they cause discomfort, urinary tract infections are usually quickly and easily treated – but it is important that they are treated promptly. A UTI will never heal itself.

UTI's are caused by bacteria entering the bladder and multiplying. Most of the time, the bacteria involved is *Escherichia coli* or, E coli. We hear a lot about E coli in the news – as a cause of food poisoning – and most strains of E.coli are harmless. In fact, they are *necessary* to the process of digestion.

But, the wrong strain in the wrong place at the wrong time…

- ***WARNING: UTI'S NEED TO BE TREATED***

UTI's sometimes come with a warning but most of the time they announce themselves with a pressing need to empty the bladder, burning or pain, and sometimes blood. As a UTI progresses, they cause fever and more general body aches.

If not treated, a UTI could continue into the urinary tract, causing a kidney infection. Again, UTI's do not simply fix themselves. They need to be treated.

As Ellen knew from past experience, the most common treatment for UTI's is an antibiotic prescribed by your doctor. The important thing to remember with any antibiotic is to use it exactly as it is prescribed and to take the full course of the medicine. Stopping early – when you are "feeling better" – leaves only the strongest bacteria in place, allowing them to multiply and to cause an even more serious infection.

Once you begin antibiotics, you should experience a dramatic improvement in a day or so. If you haven't noticed such an improvement after two days, call your doctor. The antibiotic may need to be changed.

Again, follow your doctor's instructions and finish the full course of the medicine, which will most likely be a seven to fourteen day course.

"I just hate taking antibiotics," Ellen complained when we arrived at the small bed-and-breakfast where we were going to spend the night.

While antibiotics are successful with UTI's, they are not the only treatment. D-Mannose, a type of sugar, is a very effective *natural* remedy. UTI's caused by E coli – which represent almost 90% of infections – are responsive to D-Mannose. Most of the time, D-Mannose will ease symptoms well within twenty-four hours. (As with antibiotics, even with D-Mannose, it is important to continue a course of treatment even after you feel better. In the case of D-Mannose, you should continue to take it for two to three days after the end of symptoms, just to "be sure.")

Nothing could be easier than treating yourself with D-Mannose – just add half to a full teaspoon of D-Mannose powder to a glass of water and drink it every three hours.

Simple.

It is very important to monitor your symptoms – whether you are treating your UTI with antibiotics or D-Mannose. If your symptoms don't improve, you need to be in touch with your doctor. Home remedies are often as good as, or even better, than conventional treatments. But the "bottom line" test is *whether the treatment works*. Your wellness is the goal, not a philosophical or political perspective.

I am very much an advocate for sensible and effective self-care. As I have said numerous times – and will repeat many more times – people take too many medications. Our bodies are *designed* to heal. Providing support to our bodies should not require turning ourselves into "lab rats." However, the important thing is to heal. If that can be accomplished with home remedies, great. If not, be sensible and seek medical attention!

There are about ten percent of UTI's that D-Mannose will not treat effectively. These are UTI's caused by a bacterium other than E coli. Therefore, if your symptoms don't improve within a day, call your doctor and tell her that you've treated your symptoms with D-Mannose and it wasn't successful. That information should inform your doctor's prescription decision going forward.

- ### FREQUENT UTI'S

The immediate concern with a UTI is to treat the uncomfortable symptoms as the underlying cause is addressed. However, for women who experience recurring UTI's it is most important to be focused on prevention. For any number of reasons, women who experience recurring UTI's have a urinary tract environment that favors the bacteria. Keeping the bacteria from taking hold and growing then is the primary goal.

Women – and men – suffering from frequent UTI's should adjust their daily habits so that they:

- Drink plenty of clean water. I mean *plenty* of water – 8 -10 large glasses each day.
- Use a half-teaspoon of D-Mannose once a day.
- Take a good probiotic each day to keep your E coli under control.

No one needs to suffer from the discomfort of UTI's. Taking these simple steps can do wonders to keep you from getting a UTI and, should you get one, D-Mannose can help in a hurry.

Chapter Four –
Shaving without Tears

I remember when I was a young boy. Along with my toy doctor's kit and model racers, I had a toy shaving kit. This kit consisted of a cup and brush along with a plastic double-edge razor, complete with cardboard razor blade. Sunday mornings, I would stand alongside my dad while he lathered his neck and his cheeks and I would mimic everything he did.

I can still remember how he instructed me to be careful as I brought the razor up along my neck and how he taught me to stretch the skin on my cheeks as I drew the razor along them.

When I was a young teen and received my first "real" razor – mother argued for an electric razor. I think she was worried for my safety. Dad, however, insisted that I should shave with a razor. – my dad positioned himself behind me and he guided me in the matter and manner of correctly shaving my young face. Which, for the record, did not really need to be shaved yet!

I know my sister received a similar lesson from mother about shaving her legs, although my mother kept trying to put off the lesson during many fraught dinner conversations. More than the practicalities of shaving, she felt my sister should be a bit older before she began to shave her legs.

Those days seem so long ago – not just my own childhood but a time when parents *taught* their kids such important basics as how to shave. As a result, a remarkable number of people take care of a daily task without really knowing what they're doing!

Men no longer use double-edge razors but they are bombarded with the choice of single blade, double blade, triple blade… even *four* blade. There are electric razors. All manner of shaving cream and face cream…

The choices are daunting. The frustrating thing for many men – and women – is that all these products and choices don't add up to a satisfying shave.

Now, I grant you that a close and satisfying shave is not on a plane with curing cancer or feeding the world's hungry but for men and women who start every day with razor burn or a shave that is not as close and neat as they would like it is a very important matter.

So what is a person who has not had the benefit of "Shaving 101" from their mother or father to do? What is a person to do when the various shaving products they have used don't add up to a satisfying shave?

Turn to The Compounder and The Compounder's Total Shaving Solution, of course!

- ### SHAVE WITH OIL

Unlike gels and creams, The Compounder's Total Shaving Solution is a shaving *oil* that is unconditionally guaranteed to give you the closest, smoothest, most comfortable shaving experience that you've ever had or your money back. Regardless of ethnicity, gender or skin type The Compounder's Total Shaving Solution is your solution to a great shave. Got a five o'clock shadow that shows up at three? Try The Compounder's Total Shaving Solution. I promise you, it will be the best shaving experience you've had since that plastic razor with the cardboard blade!

If you regularly experience shaving irritations like nicks and cuts, razor burns and razor bumps, The Compounder's Total Shaving Solution is for you. It will reduce those irritations to a degree you will simply not believe.

But, to quote those late night ads on television, *that's not all*. The Compounder's Total Shaving Solution is a real all-in-one shaving product. You can use it as a shaving lubricant, a pre-electric conditioner and an aftershave, and it will leave your skin soft and supple, won't clog your pores and will never, ever sting.

It packs a big punch in a small package, coming in a small bottle that travels easily and lasts a long, long time – you use **only 3 to 5 drops at a time!**

"Larry, that sounds fine and good but I like to shave in the shower..."

There is no better place to shave than in the shower. The steam and the moisture of the shower softens your facial hair and acts as a lubricant. The only trouble is, for most people, the heat and water keep their shaving gel or cream from staying in place! You won't have that problem with The Compounder's Total Shaving Solution. And unlike conventional gels, foams, lotions, and powders, it is activated by moisture and actually works best in the tub or shower. The wetter the shaving area, the better. Other than wiping the steam from your mirror, it takes care of everything.

It is absolutely ideal for shower and tub shaving.

Which brings us to those of us who shave more than our faces. Personally, I shave my head and face. The Compounder's Total Shaving

Solution is amazing. No other product comes close to this product when it comes to closeness of shave while leaving your skin soft, supple and looking and feeling *great*! No nicks. No scratches. No razor burn. Just smooth-as-a-baby's-bottom skin!

But what about those *really sensitive* areas like underarms and bikini lines?

Once again, The Compounder's Total Shaving Solution is the ideal solution to shaving woes. This all-natural, highest-quality product is made exclusively of essential oils. No water. No soaps. No alcohols. No salts. No chemicals. No preservative. No animal testing.

NO KIDDING.

Ever wonder why companies that make shaving gels and creams also make aftershave lotions? Ever wonder why they spend so many millions of dollars trying to get you to buy their products? Most of those heavily-marketed products include some or all of those ingredients! They rob your skin of its natural moisture (hence the need for aftershave lotions!) and actually contribute to dry and irritated skin.

After you've shaved with The Compounder's Total Shaving Solution, you won't need an aftershave or moisturizer because it won't make your skin dry and irritated in the first place.

It is so concentrated that you only need a few drops to do the job.

It is *clear* – allowing you to see exactly where you are shaving. No more cream and gel covering up mustaches and beards; no more guesswork when it comes to that clean bikini line!

(Helpful Hint: To minimize the unpleasant after-effects of waxing, massage a few drops of The Compounder's Total Shaving Solution into the area to be waxed, wait about 30 seconds and then proceed. You should notice a significant reduction in discomfort and redness. Try using it afterward as well to soothe and refresh your skin!)

The oils in The Compounder's Total Shaving Solution are formulated to really soften, moisturize, condition, cleanse and protect your skin both while you shave and after – leaving your skin feeling silky smooth and refreshed.

And that's not all!

The Compounder's Total Shaving Solution is elegant and efficient to use. A mere three drops per shave means that a 1/3 ounce bottle will last a man who shaves his face daily about three months. A 1.25 ounce bottle will last about a year. And, because it *naturally* moisturizes and protects your skin it effectively eliminates the need for aftershaves and moisturizers – saving money and space.

No other shaving lubricant does so much with so little!

Unlike bulky cans, it fits easily in a shaving kit or in the small cosmetic bags. No worries about "failing" the 4 ounce rule at airports! What's more, the bottle is made from recyclable plastic so it's environmentally friendly.

Try it for the shave you've been waiting for since your dad first showed you how to shave – or for the best shave you've had since you wished someone taught you how! And women… enjoy what the Total Shaving Solution does for you, leaving your legs, sensitive underarms and bikini area feeling silky soft and smooth, eliminating the need for additional lotions and creams, and it won't clog pores the way many other products do!

Chapter Five – My Throat Hurts!

- **WHY DOES MY THROAT HURT?**

Other than a belly ache, there is probably not an ailment that troubles people more – and more regularly – than a sore throat. As with any discomfort or symptom, the cause is almost always simple, straightforward and relatively benign. However, one of the real benefits of being focused on wellness and on taking care of yourself – in addition to just *feeling* better and enjoying life more – is the ability to distinguish between things that can and should be treated at home and things that require a visit to the doctor.

Just as sore throats are simple irritations, their cause is often equally simple. But some sore throats – like some belly aches – are clues to more significant conditions that need a doctor's intervention and support.

There are a number of reasons that you might have a sore throat. While infections are the most common reason for a sore throat, the soreness may also be caused by:

- A drip from your sinuses

- Pollens and molds that irritate the nose when they are inhaled may also irritate the throat
- Cat and dog dander and house dust may cause sore throats for people with allergies to them
- Dry air may create a mild sore throat with a parched feeling, especially in the mornings
- Pollutants and chemicals in the air
- Straining the voice (yelling at a sports event, for example)
- Regurgitation of stomach acids into the back of the throat
- Tumors of the throat, tongue, and larynx (voice box)

Symptoms that are mild just need to be treated, as I will discuss. However, if you experience any of the following symptoms, please see your physician to be sure that your sore throat is not more serious or a sign of a more serious problem:

- Severe or prolonged soreness
- Difficulty breathing (always seek medical care if you find you are having difficulty breathing!)
- Difficulty swallowing
- Difficulty opening your mouth
- Sore throat that is accompanied by:
- Joint pain
- Earache
- Rash
- A fever above 101°
- Blood in your saliva or phlegm

- A lump in your neck (on one or both sides)
- Hoarseness lasting more than two weeks

- **GET SOME RELIEF...**

As you can see, the cause of your sore throat may be from any number of causes. However, the important, *immediate* goal is to get you some *relief*. And the good news is that the following remedies should help you regardless of why your throat is sore.

A few commonsense actions might be helpful to anyone experiencing soreness:

- Increase your liquid intake
- Drink a cup of warm tea with honey a couple of times each day – especially at bedtime. Consider an herbal tea like Chamomile, which is particularly soothing to the throat. If you prefer not to use honey, consider using *xylitol*. It is marketed under a number of brand names. It is sweet like sugar; has no aftertaste and it is safe for diabetics and people with hypoglycemia.
- Use a humidifier in your bedroom, particularly during the winter months
- Elevate your head while you sleep – using an extra pillow should be sufficient to accomplish this
- There are also some homeopathic remedies that are helpful for sore throats. Vinceel is a good remedy that is successful for many people.

Of course, I'm also partial to some "homespun" remedies that really put the "home" into home remedies. For example, Edith, a sweet older woman who comes into The Compounder regularly, swears by an apple cider vinegar mix that her mother gave to her when she was a little girl.

"First sign of scratchiness and I take down the apple cider vinegar," she said. "I haven't had a bad sore throat since I was eight."

Nothing could be easier than Edith's solution – simply mix two tablespoons of apple cider vinegar in a glass of warm water and gargle three or more times a day. The vinegar changes the pH of the mouth and throat as well, making it a less hospitable environment for bacteria – both healing infections that have taken hold and preventing infections from starting.

A cayenne pepper solution is helpful – a sometimes more bracing! – for similar reasons. Mix half a teaspoon of cayenne pepper in a cup of hot water then allow it to cool so that it remains very warm but comfortable to gargle with. The pepper will dilate the blood vessels in your throat, helping to draw out and heal the infection.

If you want to really attack the soreness, you can add two tablespoons of apple cider vinegar to the hot cayenne pepper mix. Gargle and you can almost *feel* the healing taking place.

Of course, "you've got to know your customers" – as my grandmother used to tell me. An apple cider vinegar or cayenne pepper gargle might be palatable to most adults but if you offer it to a child you will spend most of the day trying to drag him out from under the bed! In addition, gargling is not easy for young children. So, for them I would suggest a honey and lemon juice drink. Simply mix equal parts honey and lemon juice (either fresh or in a bottle) in a glass of warm water. Sip this tasty treat slowly and feel the soreness ease!

Now, to listen to some of the older folks in the neighborhood, booze is the "special" ingredient in any of these mixtures. Ed, an older guy who works nearby, swears by the honey and lemon mixture.

"With one exception," he adds with a twinkle in his eye. "Instead of a two-part solution, make it a *three*-part solution with one part being booze."

"Booze?" I ask.

"Sure. Whiskey. Gin. Vodka. Doesn't matter. Of course," he added, "this is an *adult's only* remedy. And it should only be used when you know you won't be driving or operating any heavy machinery."

Sound advice.

A simple saltwater gargle is also helpful. Then again, there is always the "tried and true" solution for those times when you are out on the road and unable to get to a warm, soothing drink or gargle – a sucking candy.

While I don't generally recommend sugar, the sugar free candies just don't seem to work as well as sugared candy when it comes to soothing the throat. This is true of candies and cough drops – which are helpful if you have a cold or stuffy nose with your sore throat. The menthol unstuffs your nasal passages while the candy soothes your throat.

Chapter Six – What?! There Must Be Something Wrong with the Scale!

No other words strike fear in the hearts of men more than, "Honey, do I look fat is this?"

Why? Because the answer in invariably, YES. Of *course* the answer is "yes." *Everyone* looks fat in their clothes because practically everyone *is* fat. We are a nation of overweight people (apologies to those very few who are not overweight. This chapter is probably not for you in any case!) I have become convinced that makers of clothes have "re-sized" their clothes so that people can believe they are not getting bigger because they wear the "same" size they've worn for years.

Mind you, we all know that we're overweight. That's why diet books sell so incredibly well. That's why so many people use diet pills, fad diets, etc. etc. etc.

There are few better things we can do for ourselves to maintain our good health and wellness than to keep our weight under control. (Which is, I hasten to point out, a very different thing than being "skinny." While the Body Mass Index (BMI) is not a perfect measure of healthy weight, it is a reasonable one that is a useful, objective guide for knowing when too much – or too little – is too much.)

The secret to losing weight is no secret at all. Take in fewer calories than you expend. That's it. Burn more than you eat.

Simple.

Simpler said than done, actually, for most people. There are too many people who have yet to meet a donut that doesn't call their name, or a super-sized order of French fries that can be left unfinished. There are too many people for whom a jog around the park might just as well be a walk off the plank… However, if you are thinking that it is time to make peace with your bathroom scale, there are common sense methods that can help you achieve your healthy weight goals.

- ### Recommendations on Weight Loss…

These recommendations come from my friend Roy Barker, who copyrighted them in 2005. (Commentary – in italics – is mine!) Roy has an in-depth and long established background with the vitamins, minerals and health industry and has researched and experimented with many diets over a thirty-year period. He is also the author of "Safe and Easy Weight Loss", an e-book based on the Mediterranean Diet often used by those with heart conditions and those interested in a quick and safe way to shed weight.

1. Never leave home "starving." Always have a light snack before eating dinner in a restaurant, such as a piece of fruit, a glass of juice or a carrot. (*Restaurants invariably serve meals that are much too large. Make it a habit of leaving a third or half of your meal uneaten. Remember, leftovers make a great lunch the next day!*)

2. Don't go food shopping on an empty stomach! You'll be tempted to buy everything in sight. (*Actually, you will only*

be tempted to buy the very foods you <u>shouldn't</u> – potato chips, etc. That is, high calorie, high fat, and high salt foods.)

3. Don't be tempted by treats. Store them out of view, off counter-tops and as out-of-reach as possible. (*Preferably, in a neighbor's garage!*)

4. Don't eat in front of the TV. Watching the boob tube – instead of watching your plate – lulls you into overeating. Also avoid being tempted by food and snack commercials. (*Yet another good use of TiVo or DVR – skipping these tempting commercials.*)

5. Make it a rule in your house to confine your meals to the dining room or kitchen table! Never eat standing up! This leads to mindless snacking.

6. Think before you drink. Alcohol adds lots of calories, but no nutrients. Also, it weakens your willpower to avoid the wrong food choices. Hangovers can cause wicked cravings for fatty or high carbohydrate foods that can sabotage any attempt at weight loss. (*These, of course, are just the dietary reasons to <u>think</u> before you drink. There are many others.*)

7. Fill up on soup first. Begin every meal with non-cream hot soup; it forces you to eat slowly and fills you up so you won't overeat. (*Giving your stomach time to let your brain know not to feel hungry.*)

8. Take time to taste your food. Don't gobble food down! (*Remember your mother's admonition – chew your food! Doing so will cut down on your post-meal gas too.*) Rushing through your meals doesn't give your brain the time that it needs to signal your body that you are full.

9. When dining out, request sauces and low-calorie dressings on the side.

10. There is no law that requires you to finish everything on your plate.

11. Prepare a shopping list (with menu ideas in mind) and stick to the list. Avoid being tempted by bargains that grocery stores place on the outer aisles and at the back and the front of the store. The healthiest foods are usually in the long narrow aisles (*Remember, food marketers have been doing this for a long time. They know how to try and convince you to buy what they want you to buy. Be disciplined so you can buy what YOU want to buy.*)

12. Use non-stick pans to reduce the need for cooking with fat. (*Do not overheat! Some non-stick cookware is unstable at high temperatures and may release toxic fumes. Be careful. Discard any non-stick equipment that has been heated too much or that appears to be flaking or chipping.*)

13. If you must use oil, try a flavorful one like olive or sesame oil. Now remember, a little goes a long way! Make just a *spritz* of oil go even further by buying a Misto. A Misto is an aerosol can that you can fill with a good fat such as olive or canola oil.

14. A pinch of grated cheese or blue cheese will provide a flavorful kick without adding a lot of calories to a salad or grain dish.

15. If you cook in large quantities for your family, store leftovers in individual serving size containers. This is a way to practice portion control for yourself so you don't eat too much at one sitting. (*Remember, "calories per serving" is only useful if you stick to a serving size – which most of us invariably do not.*)

16. Nibbling off someone else's plate may seem harmless – but those calories do add up!

17. Drink six to eight glasses of water a day. A beverage before mealtime will also help you feel full faster and longer. Water also helps your body digest food, which is especially important now that you're eating a fiber rich diet. (*It is hard to overstate the benefits of good, clean water.*)

18. Store really tempting treats in opaque containers or silver foil – and stick them in the back of the refrigerator. (*Preferably your neighbor's refrigerator.*) Out of sight out of mind!

19. Are you stuffing yourself? If you have to loosen your belt a few notches after meals you're definitely eating too much!

20. Mashed bananas, prunes and apple sauce are great baking substitutes for fat, especially in bread, brownie and cake mixes.

21. When you choose to eat "fast food," choose wisely: skip fried foods; avoid large portions; and opt for a small hamburger.

22. Sauté foods, if possible, in chicken stock, low-sodium soy sauce or water, instead of fat.

23. When cooking, broil, bake, roast, boil or stir-fry and let the fat drain. A George Foreman grill is an excellent investment for those who want to eat meat and avoid eating the fat drippings too!

24. Sauces and soups can be thickened with a puree of potatoes instead of cream.

25. Instead of eating any product directly out of the box, pour a reasonable portion onto a plate or bowl, and put the box away. This also prevents mindless snacking.

26. If a recipe calls for 1/2 a cup of oil, cut that amount in half, your taste buds won't know the difference –but your waistline will.

27. Add spice to your life instead of fat; fresh herbs will perk up any dish without adding calories. Experiment with different ethnic foods and seasonings; they're full of flavor -- not fat.

28. Freeze leftovers immediately so you can't raid the refrigerator later.

29. Watch portion size by dishing out meals and bringing plates to the table. Don't set "bottomless" bowls and platters where they'll tempt you to reach for more, unless it's a salad or a bowl of vegetables. You can never get enough of those greens.

30. Start saving for that new outfit now! When you reach your goal weight, you can buy yourself some fashionable new clothes! (*Never, ever underestimate the value of a clear motivator. Besides, you <u>deserve</u> a reward for accomplishing your goals.*)

As you get your portion sizes and habits under control by using Roy's suggestions, you can begin to concentrate more on *what* you eat rather than just *how much* you eat. In addition to outsized portions, our diet is too often filled with fats and salts which, while appealing to our ancient dietary desires, do a great deal to diminish our wellness and good health.

John Tiniakos suggests that perhaps the answer to weight loss *and* good health can be found in a high-protein, low-saturated fat diet.

For a number of years, the "battle" in diet circles has been between the relative advantages of a high-protein, low-carbohydrate type diet versus a high-carbohydrate, low-fat diet. Recent students suggest that the high-protein, low-carb diet may be the "winner." The high-protein, low-carbohydrate diet has the greater diet induced thermogenesis (calorie burning) than a high-carbohydrate low-fat diet. (The other, much greater, method of calorie burning is, of course, exercise!)

Although diet induced thermogenesis (DIT) seems counter-intuitive, it is real. Your body's temperature increases when you digest and absorb a meal – calories are burned by this "work." You lose weight by eating! Well, kind of. You don't actually lose weight because digestion doesn't burn more calories than you are taking in. But, the more calories burned by the *process of eating* the healthier the diet. So, even though the "exercise of eating" may be the holy grail of the overeater hoping to lose weight, the truth is that there is no lazy *and* healthy way to lose weight. You simply have to work at it – mentally, psychologically, and *especially* physically.

But before you put on your running shoes and begin another diet plan, it is interesting to learn that people in certain cultures around the world whose diets contain just as much fat and carbohydrate (if not more) as the American diet manage to remain slimmer, and have much fewer occurrences of heart disease and cancer, than we do. This is particularly true in certain Mediterranean regions and in France.

Studies, particularly one done by Adam Drewnowski of the University of Michigan, have found that the French ate more foods that were higher in fat, saturated fat and cholesterol than their American counterparts, with 99% of French women's diets having saturated fat contents in excess of 10% of total daily calories.

Shocking! But what is *more* shocking is that, on average, the French are thinner and have fewer occurrences of heart disease than Americans!

Drewnowski determined that the harmful effects of the high fat content in the French diet were offset by diet diversity and variety. As he pointed out, "the low fat approach is very good but not if it comes at the expense of dietary variety." Of course, USDA recommendations call for variety. But just one in ten men and one in sixteen women consume food from all five food groups the USDA recommends.

In addition, Drewnowski found that the French tend to have more active lifestyles than we do.

Similarly, the Mediterranean diet is high in fat, but more diverse than the American diet. So too, certain Mediterranean people, particularly from the Greek island of Crete, had fewer cases of heart disease and were thinner than Americans.

Studies of the Mediterranean diet have concluded that much of the good health benefit of the diet comes from the essential fatty acids that can be found in foods in the diet. By studying the different health outcomes based on diet (and not just on foods,) scientists have concluded that both the French and Mediterranean diets consist of more foods containing omega-3s than the American diet does, whereas ours contains more foods containing omega-6s.

The biology and chemistry can be daunting but the bottom line is that the relative amount of these essential fatty acids is key. The primary reason we have a lower intake of omega-3s is because we eat an incredible amount of processed food. Food processing *as a process* removes the majority of the omega-3 content from food.

The French and Mediterranean diets are more abundant in whole foods, fresh fruits and vegetables. Absent food processing, their intake of omega-3s is considerably higher than ours.

These various studies make clear that fat content alone is not determinative when it comes to weight gain and health. These two cultures manage to stay healthier and slimmer than we do while eating foods that contain high fat, carbohydrate and protein contents. The difference is that the French and Mediterranean diets contain more unrefined foods; they consist of foods from all food groups and have more variety.

As a result, the people in these places tend to be both thinner *and* healthier despite eating more foods that would *seem* to contribute to weight gain. Of course, as I've mentioned, they are also more physically active than we are. So, it is time to lace up your sneakers and walk – or jog – to the supermarket for a new supply of fresh, wholesome food.

Isn't it time you won the argument with your bathroom scale?

Isn't it time for you to take care of your health *and* your waistline?

Section Three – Healthy Choices

Introduction – Wellness is a Choice

The more we learn about biology, the more we come to appreciate the truth that, to some extent, genetics are destiny. Why do some people smoke every day of their adult lives and live to be ninety-five while the vast majority of us lose years of life by smoking? Why do some people eat to their heart's desire without gaining weight while others of us merely *look* at food and gain weight? Why do some of us get cancers that grow so violently and relentlessly while others survive multiple bouts of cancer?

The answers to these questions remain to be fully answered. What our current understandings suggest is that our genetic make-up has a great deal to do with these things. But, while genetics may prove to be ultimately determinative in certain ways, we absolutely know that we have direct control over a myriad of factors that contribute not only to our health but to our greater, and more important, wellness.

We know that obesity contributes to all sorts of health deficits. While genetics may determine our overall body type, *we* have control of how we best inhabit that body type. Remember, nothing is more beautiful or sexy than a person who is comfortable and healthy in their own skin!

We know that we are too often subject to dangerous air, and that soot, car exhaust and factory exhaust contributes to respiratory ailments. We ask a great deal of the filtering systems in our lungs, overwhelming them with the ills of our environment. Our biology may determine our individual strength in filtering these pollutants but the *decision* to smoke or not smoke is the single greatest determinant for healthy lungs and lifelong breathing.

Someone whose parents died prematurely of heart disease is statistically at greater risk for heart disease. But choosing a healthy diet and active lifestyle will not only maximize the years that genetics allots you, but it will also maximize your enjoyment of the years of your life.

Too much of our lives are "quantified" – we measure everything. How much we earn. How big our houses are. How many cars we drive. Our blood pressure readings. Our cholesterol levels. Our weight. The number of calories we consume. The number of miles we run. All of these "numbers" may be important and may contribute to good health but they do not add up to our sense of wellness.

Wellness is *qualitative*. It is a measure, yes, but not one easily defined.

When you proactively take care of your good health, you automatically contribute to your sense of wellness because you are not only taking care of your biology, you are taking control of your own life and nothing is as satisfying and enriching as being in control of the things that are important to us.

Chapter One –
What "They" Don't Want You to Know about Vitamins

If we all lived a perfectly healthy lifestyle and ate a complete, varied and healthy diet we would avoid a great many illnesses and maladies. It is a monumental understatement to say simply, We don't. Willie Sutton, the bank robber, was once asked why he robbed banks. His answer? *Because that's where the money is.* The medical and food industries have translated our bad choices and habits into incredible profits. Just as Willie Sutton robbed banks because that's where the money was, these industries *depend* on our bad habits and choices to make money.

Beware of the advice of those who profit from the answer!

Food processing strips food of essential components. As a result, even those of us who try make healthy food choices are well served to supplement our diets with vitamins and minerals. It should come as no surprise then that industries that profit from our ill health might suggest that simple, and inexpensive, ways of getting what we need for good health might challenge the efficacy of vitamins and minerals.

I was troubled but not shocked to see a November 9th, 2008 Yahoo news report written by Marilynn Marchione, an Associated

Press Medical Writer, proclaim, "Vitamin Pills Don't Prevent Heart Disease."

Yahoo is a credible news source and the AP is even more so. Still, it seemed to me to be a fairly bold statement. So, instead of accepting it on face value, I decided to take a closer look. The study the headline referred to consisted of 14,461 male doctors, fifty years old or older, including 5% who had heart disease at the time of the study.

The men in the study were given either vitamin C, vitamin E, both, or a dummy pill. After eight years the researchers determined that there were *no differences* in the rates of heart attacks, stroke, or heart-related deaths.

At first glance, this conclusion seems like a powerful finding. However, the boldface conclusion fails to account for some of the very important subtleties of the study. For example, one could – and should – question not only what vitamins were part of the study but also what dosage was administered. In evaluating the study, the dosages of the study were 500 mg of vitamin C and 400 IU of vitamin E.

The daily recommended amount (RDA) of vitamin C – as established by the U.S. Government around the time of World War II – is about 65 mg. Based on that recommendation, 500 mg would seem ample. But Dr. Linus Pauling, the physicist turned researcher, suggested daily doses in the *thousands* of milligrams. In the early 60s, Dr. Pauling suggested a 3,000 mg dose. A few short years later, he had increased his recommendation to around 18,000 mg! Compared to 18,000 mg, 500 mg seems fairly piddling. In fact, it is only about 3% of the dose Pauling and others recommend for heart protection.

The question the study does not even pose is what the threshold dose of vitamin C! Imagine if a similar study was conducted on penicillin, one in which a dose only 3% of the effective dose was used. We would see headlines proclaiming the ineffectiveness of penicillin to combat disease!

And the headlines would be right... but incomplete. What they *should* proclaim is that penicillin is ineffective *at the tested dose*. Likewise, the AP report should have made clear that vitamin C was not effective at the dose tested. However, as long as prominent and credible researchers and scientists claim that greater doses are safe and effective, the more absolute statement should be muted.

It should go without saying that the dose of vitamin E under study was also much lower than is being suggested by modern researchers.

It is reasonable to test a dose greater than the recommended daily intake levels. But it is equally reasonable to remember that the RDA is a very small dose and was established to provide the *absolute minimum* required to prevent serious, adverse health consequences and death. In addition, the RDA's were established during a time when food processing was still in its infancy and the food most people actually ate was far more nutritious than it is today. In other words, when supplements were less necessary.

To truly test a supplement's efficacy in fighting disease, it seems to me that a researcher would use dosages suggested by some of the pioneering researchers like Pauling. Unless, of course, the researcher wanted to show *minimal* effect. Then it would make perfect sense to choose a minimal dose but one that could be easily justified based on "common knowledge" and "consensus."

To test 500 mg of vitamin C when Pauling recommends 18,000 mg makes clear the study's intention – to discredit the use of vitamins in disease prevention. After all, a "reasonable" person would be reasonable in concluding from the results of the study that vitamins are basically useless. Or, in the words of some, "expensive urine additives."

Which is the exact conclusion that Big Pharma has been promoting for years. But remember my warning: Beware of the advice of people who profit from the answer. The pharmaceutical industry has a vested interest in discrediting the benefit of inexpensive, readily available vitamins that can accomplish what its very expensive drugs purport to do.

If the vitamins work, they lose money. Hence, it is beneficial to them to make "clear" that vitamins don't work.

And lest anyone even *think* that maybe, possibly vitamins may be able to do what some of us suggest that they do, the pharmaceutical industry goes even further than claiming that they are ineffective; they go so far as to suggest that they are *dangerous*. Too much (whatever *that* is!) vitamin C can harm you! Too much vitamin E "builds up" in your body!

Big Pharma has one goal and one goal only – to make sure that you take their (very expensive) drugs to combat disease. In this goal, they seem to have the full support of the FDA. The FDA makes clear its contention that the *only* legal cure for any disease is a regulated drug.

Checkmate.

Sort of. It is, actually, simply flawed, circular reasoning. It is, in short, a con job! The study and its much-trumpeted conclusions are flawed. The dosing is subject to significant challenge. Such a significant flaw cannot help but raise doubts about every other aspect of the study. All other aspects of the study become mere "window dressing" when fundamental premises are flawed.

That impressive study group? Irrelevant. (Note: there is no mention of how the researchers handled the 5% of participants who had heart disease at the beginning of the study. Was their outcome, even at the low doses, different from the rest of the participants?)

The report's suggestion that **taking vitamin E is potentially dangerous?** Come on! The report claims a 74% greater risk of bleeding strokes in those participants who were taking the vitamin E. If I was a "reasonable" reader of the report's conclusions, that would sure sound like a significant difference. I'd be willing to wager that the people who sponsored the research intended it to look that way.

But, **what are the real facts?**

The groups that used vitamin E recorded 39 strokes as compared to 23 in the group that was NOT taking vitamin E. A difference of 16 cases. On first glance, that is *a lot*. But *statistically* it is not nearly as significant as it seems. If half the men in the study received vitamin E and the other half didn't, then the statistical difference is really 16/7230, or 0.22%.

0.22%? That's it?

Yep. And, I think anyone can see that 0.22% is *a lot* different than 74%. And a lot less frightening. Of course, the larger number grabs the most attention. But the larger number is deceptive. So too are the other instances of dramatically high numbers. In total, 62 of the participants experienced a stroke – 0.4% of the study population. (The overall incidence of stroke in white people was 0.4%, 0.6% for blacks, and 0.679% for American Indians. That is, the incidence of stroke in this study is actually *below* the overall incidence reported for the general population. (*source:* American Heart Association)

In my reading of the study, I do not think the actual data – versus the exaggerated interpretation of the data – supports the contention that vitamin E poses a risk. Or, to make it more personal, will this report change my own habit of taking vitamin C or vitamin E every day? Not a chance.

Why would I "blindly" engage in such activity if this study PROVED that it was useless and possibly – probably! – dangerous to do so? Simple. From my perspective, **the study failed to prove anything.** What's more, it didn't even address a couple of very significant realities: Our food supply is severely depleted in nutrients. In fact, the nutrient content of today's produce is less than a third of what it was only 40 years ago.

Supplements are necessary.

Supplements help promote health and reduce illness. And wellness is the necessary result of these things. When it comes to assessing the behaviors that contribute to your good health and well-being, you need to factor in the *source* of the information that you are receiving and then make your decisions accordingly.

If Big Pharma and the food processing industry are trumpeting the results of a study… beware!

Chapter Two – Smoking and the <u>REAL</u> "Little Blue Pill"

At The Compounder, we regularly compound a prescription preparation for erectile dysfunction (ED). It is administered by injection and, judging by the numbers of refill requests we get, the treatment works just dandy. However, it is not the treatment of ED that is of particular interest to me just now. What is of interest to me is an observation I've made in filling prescriptions for the compound – just how many of the men who come in for the medication smell of cigarette smoke.

At The Compounder, we do not fill prescriptions for the more famous, and popular, oral ED medications – Cialis and Viagra – so I couldn't say either anecdotally or accurately if those men also smell of cigarette smoke, but I would hazard a guess that a good many of them *do*. Which suggests just one downside to cigarette smoke, albeit a significant one!

An erection is a brilliant example of biological engineering at its best, engineering that is often not well understood. The reason for much of this misunderstanding begins with a misconception of the penis itself. To wit, the penis is *not* a muscle, which explains why it is less "controllable" than other muscles in our body and why, in truth, it sometimes seems to have a "mind of its own." It is an organ. Most men don't give this distinction much thought until they find themselves in the position of wanting to exert control over their penis as they might over any muscle in their body. It is then that they fully appreciate that getting an erection is not like flexing a bicep.

The penis actually operates (in an erection sense) by a passive use of pressure. When a man becomes aroused, the arteries leading into the penis dilate, bringing blood rushing into the penis. At the same time, the veins constrict, forcing the blood into the corpus cavermosa – elongating and becoming firm. That is, becoming erect.

If the arteries leading to the penis do not dilate or, for any reason, restrict the amount of blood coming into the penis, ED will result.

When you were eighteen years old, the mere suggestion of something arousing (and recognizing that to an eighteen year old "something arousing" could be just about *anything*,) might cause an erection and this process worked flawlessly. However, at forty-five? At fifty-five? Maybe not so much.

What changed?

The greatest change is most likely life experience, bringing with it a maturing sensibility as to what is "arousing." But that does not explain why the "machinery" doesn't work as well as it used to. The fact is, like just about every other aspect of our biology, the "machinery" has been designed to last a lifetime. If it doesn't then something has broken down in the mechanics and what that "something" is has everything to do with why I smell cigarette smoke on so many of the men who come in for the compound.

A study done at Tulane University in New Orleans looked at men in China between the ages 35 and 74 who did not have signs or symptoms of cardiovascular disease. They discovered that there was a significant and direct statistical link between the number of cigarettes a man smoked and the likelihood that he would experience ED. The researchers concluded that of the men with ED, almost 25% of the cases could be directly attributed to cigarette smoking. And, of perhaps greater note, the *more* they smoked, the more profound their ED.

I can imagine the smokers reading this just groaning in frustration. What *else* can we blame on cigarettes? Well, the connection between cigarettes and ED is actually a very straightforward and clear one.

The average cigarette delivers about 1 mg of nicotine. Among its many properties, nicotine is a vasoconstrictor. It causes them to constrict, to become smaller and tighter. This tightening limits the ability of the arteries, the vessels that carry oxygenated blood to the body's tissues and cells, to do so effectively.

It is no wonder that the first people to suffer from – if not complain of – cold fingers and toes during those delightful winter walks are cigarette smokers. They also tend to get short of breath sooner.

Nicotine is a seductive and powerful drug. It crosses the blood-brain barrier and exerts its influence on nearly every cell in the body. It triggers the release of epinephrine and norepinephrine, hormones which increase blood pressure, heart rate, and breathing rates. These two powerful hormones cause the body to release stores of fat and cholesterol into the blood. They are associated with an increase in blood glucose levels.

These cascading events happen *each and every time* you smoke a cigarette.

When we are young, we are able to filter the nicotine from our systems more effectively. However, as we age, our livers lose some of their effectiveness and our ability to get the nicotine out of our bodies declines. (The use of alcohol – a frequent companion of the social smoker – increases the demand on the liver to filter the blood.) It is no wonder that male smokers who regularly consume alcohol often find themselves at the mercy of ED. Oh the irony! Alcohol, the social lubricant and sexual disinhibitor of their youth is exacting its revenge.

And the poor, middle-aged smoker? If he is able to overcome his shame, he searches in earnest for a "cure" – often in the form of a "little blue pill."

Drug manufacturers are thrilled by this dynamic. Rather than examining the causes of ED and working in concert to eliminate them, modern medicine has – to tremendous profit – sought a "fix" by finding ways to counteract the effects of blood vessels that have been constricted by nicotine and alcohol.

The logic is as simple as it is troubling. A drug got you into this mess. A drug must get you out of it.

We seek a return to our "youth" when our bodies and our bad habits had not yet turned against us. But the reality is, no one can make themselves younger. No medication. No surgery. No hormone. Nothing. Wellness suggests that a life well lived and enjoyed means always being comfortable in your own skin. There are things we can control – like our lifestyle choices – and things we can't – like our age. It would seem reasonable that a man who suffers from ED would pause and consider the behavior that has resulted in his distress. But no. How much easier to simply pop a pill and *viola!* an erection! Wonder of wonders! Miracle of miracles!

Also, this preparation must be injected directly into the penis… However, I must confess, I cringe at the mere thought of injecting anything directly into the penis… certainly when there is a reasonable alternative available, which is cutting back on tobacco and alcohol. Imagine making a lifestyle change that will not only minimize the possibility of ED but that will also improve your cardiac and pulmonary health. How is it that people don't embrace the change? The answer is because they are addicted to nicotine.

That's right. We don't generally use a term like this to describe cigarette smokers but smokers who have tried to quit can attest to the difficulty they have. Tobacco/nicotine grips them in a tight vise. The fact is, nicotine is one of the most addictive substances we know about. That it is present in a "legal" product does not minimize its addictive properties.

I have visited people dying from end-stage lung cancer, or throat cancer who continue to smoke, *unable* to stop. Kicking the smoking habit is one of the most difficult things to do – but the benefits of doing so are so monumental that everyone should be motivated to do so.

What I would like you to remember in this chapter, however, is not that nicotine is an addictive substance or that tobacco causes all sorts of profound deficits in the human body. It is that ED is *not* the result of a drug deficiency. As such, its "solution" should not be sought in a drug.

Big Pharma has made billions of dollars by creating new diseases, diseases that, conveniently, they have a pill for. There isn't a human condition for which Big Pharma will not create a disease if it believes there is money to be made in treating that disease.

Those of us focused on wellness try to remember that causes have effects. If we are not happy with the effects, we would be wise to examine the causes and make some fundamental changes in our lives and behavior.

Chapter Three – Counting to Ten; the "Ten Day" Rule

When I was a boy and I would get mad about something, which invariably meant I would say something I later regretted, my mother always counseled patience. "Count to ten before you say anything," she advised.

Who knew that "ten" would turn out to be such a foundational number?

I can't say that I always followed my mother's wise advice but it occurred to me again a number of years ago when I found myself on the business end of a spiked volleyball… back in the early 1990s, I was in the middle of a very competitive game of volleyball when I found myself at the net face-to-face with a very formidable – and tall! – opponent. This one rally was very intense, with several very dramatic digs keeping it alive. Then, the setter floated a perfect set at the net in front of me. I went up for the block. The hitter soared higher and higher, bringing his mighty hand down against the volleyball and sending it directly down into my face.

Before I knew it, I was flat on my back. I really have no recollection if the ball bounced up off my face and remained alive or if it simply skittered to the side of the court. I do, however, have a very vivid memory of the sting on my face and the solicitous concern of my teammates, all gathered around and nodding.

"Gonna have a hell of a shiner there, Larry."

"Just help me find my contact," I grumbled, as I clamored to my knees and began to slide the palms of my hands over the court.

The next morning, with my reddened eye and shiner, I headed to my ophthalmologist to make sure that the damage was only to my pride. He carefully examined me and then announced that everything would be just fine in ten days.

"Ten days?" I asked.

He nodded. "Ten days."

Sure enough. Ten days later, the redness and swelling were gone. At nine days, there was still soreness. But ten days? Viola! I was, of course, thrilled that my injury was healed. But I was intrigued by my doctor's predictive powers. He had sounded so certain. How had he known?

A few weeks later, I saw my doctor at a dinner party. As soon as I spotted him, I hurried over to him. "How did you know?" I asked him.

He looked at me. "How did I know what?"

"That my eye would be completely healed in ten days," I went on insistently.

He chuckled. "Larry," he said, resting his hand on my shoulder, "it's *always* ten days." Then he turned back to the conversation he was having before I'd rushed over to ask him my question.

"Hmm," I whistled, standing there by myself, thinking. It's *always* ten days. That was when I thought of my mother's words for the first time in a long, long while.

Of course, there are a few "magic" numbers. Three jumps to mind. Three is a recurring number in all sorts of places, from religion to fairy tales to engineering designs. Three is, in many ways, a perfect number. The source of that significance could also be practical. After all, a triangle is the strongest physical structure.

Four is another magic number, perhaps due to the "four" directions.

Ten is certainly a powerful number in Western culture. After all, our entire number system is based on the number ten. But how did that give it a predictive quality? Yet, I could not deny that, in my experience, most medical-type problems resolve themselves in about ten days – unless something is seriously wrong.

Too often we forget that our bodies are remarkable self-healing entities. Big Pharma has been very successful at convincing us that we *need* the assistance of all sorts of medications not only to get better but to maintain good health. That simply is not true. Even when we get sick, our bodies generally heal themselves, given sufficient time and care (which might mean staying in bed to rest and drinking extra fluids!)

As my mother counseled in a different context, patience goes a long way when it comes to our good health. We are so often in a rush to *take something* or to see the doctor. There is an old adage about the common cold that's worth remembering: If your doctor prescribes something for you, the cold will clear up in about seven days. Of course, if you don't go to the doctor and "tough it out" your cold will likely take a week to clear up.

Our bodies are really very good at healing themselves – almost all of the time.

Too many people rush to the doctor or the emergency room at the first sign of symptoms. They want the latest and best – and, often, the most costly – treatment. And they want it *now*. However, unless your symptoms suggest a potentially life-threatening illness (shortness of breath, chest pain, sudden weakness or paralysis on one side of your body, etc.) the very best treatment might actually be time, not drugs.

Some herbs. Some vitamins. Probiotics. And a few days. Say about ten.

As my mother taught me, count to ten – days. You should be back to your good old self by then.

It makes good, intuitive sense. If your symptoms suddenly appear, you can be relatively confident that they will resolve themselves in a week to ten days. If, after ten days the symptoms linger, or have gotten worse, it might be a good time to get to a doctor. Waiting ten days is probably a sign of good wellness. Waiting longer than that if symptoms don't go away is probably a sign of denial – and of something that does require medical intervention. For example, I recently saw a video about Inflammatory Breast Cancer (IBC), a serious condition that demands prompt attention. The video related one very sad story about a woman who visited a doctor about the sudden onset of her symptoms.

The doctor told the woman that what she had was probably a bug bite and that they'd look at it again "in six months." Tragically, she had IBC. The waiting reduced her chance for healing. Six months was too long. For her, the "ten day rule" would have been a life saver. If she would have acted promptly and found help after ten days, her outcome might have been very different.

Time was not going to heal this disease.

Be wise about your self-care. Be patient and caring about yourself. But don't wait too long. Time is your friend when it heals. It is your enemy if you delay too long. There are times when the ten day rule will fail. Some sudden symptoms need to be dealt with *immediately* and, of course; serious injuries should be evaluated right away.

Chapter Four – Water, Water Everywhere....

Only oxygen is more essential to life than water. We are made up primarily of water. We need water. Yet we don't truly understand or respect water. In particular, we don't have a sensible understanding of distilled water. For some reason, it has been shadowed by controversy and misunderstandings. Myths and fallacies affect our thinking about it. Sadly, to our disadvantage.

Let's think about water, specifically drinking water, for a moment. Most of us get our drinking water and our cooking water from the faucets in our house. Of course, this water comes from various natural sources – lakes, streams, rivers, etc. This natural water is treated at local water treatment plants where it is generally chlorinated to kill harmful bacteria. Water treatment is essential in making drinking water "drinkable." However, many harmful pollutants and bacteria are not removed in this manner.

Distilled water has been heated to boiling so that the water becomes steam, or water vapor. The steam is then "re-condensed" into its pure liquid form, leaving the impurities behind. Distilled water contains no solids, debris, toxins or other contaminants.

That's it. That's what distilled water is – 100% water. H_2O. So why all the fuss? Let's look at some of the myths about distilled water and try to make sense of them – and set them straight!

Myth #1: Distillation takes all the beneficial minerals out of water

If I had a penny for every time someone made this claim… First, this statement only has significance if non-distilled water *has* beneficial minerals, "beneficial" being the operative word here. Distillation kills and removes bacteria, viruses, cysts, as well as, heavy metals, radionuclides, organics, inorganics, and particulates. And yes, it will remove minerals, which fall under a category of inorganic contaminants. The big question is whether or not the minerals in water are beneficial or not.

All of our minerals are derived from the food we eat: fresh fruits, vegetables, meat, poultry, grains, nuts, and dairy products. The minerals in water are so scant that in Boston, MA for example, one would have to drink 676 8 oz. glasses of tap water to obtain the Recommended Daily Allowance (RDA) of calcium. That same person would have to drink 1,848 8 oz. glasses to get RDA of magnesium, 848 8 oz. glasses to get RDA of iron, and 168,960 8 oz. glasses to obtain the RDA of phosphorus… you get the idea.

With most people hard-pressed to drink even the recommended 8 glasses of water a day, it seems misplaced to concern ourselves with such low levels of mineral content.

Distilled water is pure water. Distillation removes the broadest range of contaminants over any other point of use (POU) system.

Myth #2: Distilled water leaches minerals from your body

What an image! Water actually *taking minerals away* from your body! This myth implies that because distilled water is so pure, drinking it will leach minerals from your body, thereby robbing you of good health and nutrition. This is so ridiculous as to be insulting. The national best-selling health and diet book, "Fit for Life II: Living Health," by Harvey & Marilyn Diamond, addresses this myth directly.

"Distilled water has an inherent quality. Acting almost like a magnet, it picks up rejected, discarded, and unusable minerals and, assisted by the blood and the lymph, carries them to the lungs and kidneys for elimination from the body. The statement that distilled water leaches minerals from the body has no basis in fact. It doesn't leach out minerals that have become part of the cell structure. It can't and won't. It collects only minerals that have already been rejected or excreted by the cells...To suggest that distilled water takes up minerals from foods so that the body derives no benefit from them is absurd."

Myth #3: Long, continued drinking of distilled water could cause tooth decay

Once again, "follow the money." Don't take advice from people who will profit from it. I saw this claim in the product literature of a national water filter company. Shame on them! This company mounts a false campaign to justify selling water filters.

Distillation does remove fluoride but there is no proof that this will damage teeth.

Myth #4: Distilled water tastes bland or "flat"

This is probably the most prevalent myth about distilled water and can be addressed in several ways.

First, in the past, the original distillers did not incorporate any pre- or post-carbon filtration. Straight, distilled water without the use of any pre- or post-carbon filtration sometimes has a "steamy" or slightly "off" taste. Carbon filtration solves this by going through the following process: chlorine, odors, sediment, and other organic contaminants are pre-filtered from tap or well water before it reaches the boiling tank of the distiller. After the steam is condensed into distilled water it is then passed through a carbon post-filter to remove any potential gases or volatile organic contaminants (VOCs) that might have escaped during the boiling process. Not using a post-filter in the past might have produced an off taste in distilled water, due to VOCs.

The carbon post-filter is most important because it acts as a "polishing filter" to clean up any volatile gases, which can produce an off-taste that may have escaped during the boiling process.

The more probable reason people assign this myth to distilled water is because they are accustomed to drinking chlorinated or well water, high in iron content. What they are tasting is the *absence* of these contaminates.

"Taste" is the primary reason consumers give for purchasing bottled water – to the tune of $4 billion a year. Many consumers have been led to believe that you need minerals in water to give it its taste. In truth, it is oxygen that gives water its taste. Water shouldn't have a taste or a metallic after bite.

Try either a cold or room temperature glass of freshly made distilled water and taste the difference for yourself... It's delicious.

Another reason for the "flat taste" may have to do with the fact that virtually all distilled water is purchased in the store, bottled in cheap, plastic containers. Water is the universal solvent, whatever it touches it will pick up. Distilled water being virtually 100% contaminant free might leach plastic tastes into the water from the inferior bottle it is being stored in. Besides glass, consider buying bottles made from Lexan that won't give off any plastic tastes or odors.

Myth # 5: Distilled water isn't effective against organic chemicals

VOCs are organic chemicals that have lower boiling points than tap water. Therefore, if VOCs are present, they will vaporize before the water reaches the boiling point. That is why many distillers today use a volatile gas vent - a pin hole in the top of the condensing coils to vent off any unwanted gases. VOCs that do escape this vent are trapped by the carbon post-filter. (Carbon pre-treatment will remove most chlorine and VOCs.) In cases of manual distillers, only post carbon filtration is used and is sufficient in removing VOCs and unwanted gases.

Distillation without carbon filtration is not as effective in removing VOCs by itself. Combining carbon filtration with distillation will boost removal rates to greater than 99% under normal conditions.

Myth # 6: Distillers are expensive to run

Home distillers require about 3 kilowatt hours to make 1 gallon of distilled water. The average kilowatt hour of electricity in the Unites States is about 7.8 cents, that's around 24 cents to make 1 gallon.

Is a quarter per gallon too much to pay for pure distilled water made fresh in your home?

Just compare: Distilled water from the store costs between 89 cents and $1.29 per gallon. Making your own distilled water is *very* cost effective. Why buy the milk when you can have the cow at home.

Maintenance of a distiller is changing pre- and/or post-carbon filters about every 6 - 12 months and periodically draining out the residue left over from the boiling process.

Conclusion

These myths have plagued distilled water for too long – to the detriment of the beneficial effects of drinking distilled water. There is a definite need for the home distiller market in the industry and consumers have a right to know the correct facts concerning distilled water.

And perhaps they will convince you to distill your own water!

CONCLUSION

Find a nice, comfortable place to sit down. Settle yourself in. Take a nice, slow breath. Now, another. Close your eyes and let your body relax.

Do you feel how easily the air glides into and out of your lungs? How easily your thoughts calm when you relax? What you do not feel is the magnificent process of your blood flowing through your arteries, picking up rich oxygen from your lungs and then carrying it to all the cells, tissues and organs of your body. What you do not feel is the constant process by which your body's temperature is maintained, along with your heart rate and blood pressure. You do not feel the constant regeneration of cells and tissues, replenishing your body second after second, minute after minute. You do not feel the hormones and chemicals coursing through your body, taking care of the myriad of functions necessary for you to live and thrive. You do not feel your immune system "beating up" on foreign bodies long before you feel the slightest symptom of illness – and often taking care of the intruder without your ever feeling sick at all!

Relax.

In this book, I have tried to communicate that first and foremost your body's natural state is _wellness_. While it is true that our systems sometimes go haywire, causing disease and discomfort, our bodies are actually designed to be healthy and, should we become unhealthy, to heal themselves!

Bear in mind, I am not some "flaky" and "feely-touchy" guy. I'm a scientist. I have studied chemistry and biology. I have been compounding pharmaceuticals for a long, long time. I *value* the great benefit that modern medicine bestows upon those of us requiring it. However, I have learned that *most of us* don't require it. Most of us need to listen to our bodies and to take advantage of simple, body-supporting methods to ease what ails us.

We need to stop "making up" diseases so that pharmaceutical companies can sell us "cures" for those diseases and start listening to our bodies. More importantly, we have to begin to behave in ways that support our body systems, not break them down.

Wellness is our natural state. Maintaining it requires healthy eating and living. When our bodies do go "out of balance" rather than look to a "quick fix" in a pill, we need to seek a solution that is a bit closer to the source of our problem.

If smoking cigarettes contributes to your ED, stop smoking. Don't just add another pill to the mix. If you feel that you are suffering from bad breath, make sure your digestion is in order. If you are overweight, adjust your eating habits before taking pills or, worse, going "under the knife."

I have a good friend who often reminds me that, "the correct answer is generally the simplest one."

When it comes to our health, we have too often complicated our understandings. Good health – wellness – is really nothing more than the simple, common sense care of yourself. Whether you have a cold, a UTI, bad breath, ED, or a sore throat the remedy, the way back to balance, is generally simple and straightforward. More often than not, it simply means doing the things that allow your body to heal itself.

Drink clean water and take your vitamins. Eat well. And use common sense to take care of the minor slights and injuries that the world visits upon you. And find yourself a kind and caring compounding pharmacist!

Take another slow breath. Open your eyes. The world looks brighter now. Raise a glass and toast your wellness with some fresh water!

Be well!

There are countless people who make a significant impact on our lives. I'd be hard pressed to recall most of them. There are people today who influence my thoughts and actions. These are good people who are not influenced by the status quo. They are not actually rebels in the field of health care, but they recognize that the standard approach is often not the best. These are the people who would think twice - or three times - before jumping off a bridge "just because their friends did it".

I am inserting this brief list of people I turn to today, not as an endorsement, but as a way of thanking them for their positive influence on my life and the lives of others.

Dr. Martin Plotkin http://www.wellnessconceptsllc.net/index.html

- Dr. Jeffrey Dach http://www.drdach.com/
- Dr. Hyla Cass http://www.cassmd.com/
- Dr. Jonathan Wright http://www.tahomaclinic.com/
- Dr. West Conner http://www.medicinecoach.com/
- Caroline Sutherland http://www.carolinesutherland.com/index.cfm
- Dr. Melody Hart http://www.hartcenter.com/
- Amy Biank http://www.amybiank.com/Welcome.html
- Dr. Steven Ayre http://www.contemporarymedicine.com

Testimonial

Larry is one of those rare breeds when it comes to health care. He has perfected his craft through years of knowledge, study, and hands-on experience. Most medical professionals will simply hand you a pill for your problem, not "The Compounder." As a fellow pharmacist and "rogue," I've seen the forward thinking trail that Larry has left for us...a trail cut with scientific knowledge, grandma's wisdom, and common sense when it comes to health. You will gain much insight from reading this book, as I did. Larry knows his stuff and when I have a question, I call on Larry.

West Conner PharmD
http://www.MedicineCoach.com

www.ingramcontent.com/pod-product-compliance
Lightning Source LLC
Chambersburg PA
CBHW020013050426
42450CB00005B/449